Computed Tomography of the Spine

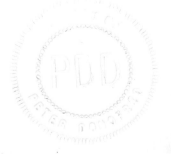

Contemporary Issues in Computed Tomography Volume 2

SERIES EDITOR

Stanley S. Siegelman, M.D.
Professor of Radiology
The Johns Hopkins University School of Medicine
Director of Diagnostic Radiology
The Johns Hopkins Hospital
Baltimore, Maryland

Volumes Already Published

Vol. 1 Computed Tomography of the Pancreas, Stanley S. Siegelman, Editor

Forthcoming Volumes in the Series

Vol. 3 Computed Tomography of the Kidneys and Adrenals, Stanley S. Siegelman, Stanford Goldman, and Olga M. Gatewood, Editors

Vol. 4 Computed Tomography of the Chest, Stanley S. Siegelman, Editor

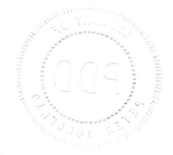

Computed Tomography of the Spine

Edited by

Victor M. Haughton, M.D.

Professor of Radiology
Department of Radiology
The Medical College of Wisconsin
Milwaukee, Wisconsin

CHURCHILL LIVINGSTONE
NEW YORK, EDINBURGH, LONDON, AND MELBOURNE
1983

Distributed in the United Kingdom by Churchill Livingstone, Robert Stevenson House, 1-3 Baxter's Place, Leith Walk, Edinburgh EH1 3AF and by associated companies, branches and representatives throughout the world.

First published 1983

Printed in USA

ISBN 0-443-08253-7

7 6 5 4 3 2 1

Library of Congress Cataloging in Publication Data
Main entry under title:

Computed tomography of the spine.

    (Contemporary issues in computed tomography; 2)
    Bibliography: p.
    Includes index.
    1. Spine—Diseases—Diagnosis.   2. Spine—
Radiography.   3. Tomography.   I. Haughton, Victor M.
II. Series.   [DNLM: 1. Spine—Radiography.
2. Tomography, X-Ray computed. W1 C0769MQK v. 2 /
WE 725 C738]
RD768.C65   1983   617'.56   83-2080
ISBN 0-443-08253-7

Contributors

Guillermo F. Carrera, M.D.
Associate Professor of Radiology and Orthopaedic Surgery, Department of Radiology, The Medical College of Wisconsin, Chief, Musculoskeletal Radiology, Milwaukee Regional Medical Center, Milwaukee, Wisconsin

David L. Daniels, M.D.
Assistant Professor of Radiology, Department of Radiology, The Medical College of Wisconsin, Milwaukee, Wisconsin

John P. Grogan, M.D.
Instructor of Radiology, Department of Radiology, The Medical College of Wisconsin, Milwaukee, Wisconsin

Victor M. Haughton, M.D.
Professor of Radiology, Department of Radiology, The Medical College of Wisconsin, Milwaukee, Wisconsin

Johan Johansen, M.D.
Fellow in Radiology, The Medical College of Wisconsin, Milwaukee, Wisconsin

Patrick A. Turski, M.D.
Assistant Professor of Radiology, Department of Radiology, University of Wisconsin-Madison, Clinical Science Center, Madison, Wisconsin

Patrick R. Walsh, M.D.
Assistant Professor of Neurosurgery, Department of Neurosurgery, The Medical College of Wisconsin, Milwaukee, Wisconsin

Alan L. Williams, M.D.
Associate Professor of Radiology, Department of Radiology, The Medical College of Wisconsin, Milwaukee, Wisconsin

Preface

Suspected spine pathology is presently one of the most important indications for CT scanning, both in terms of how frequently radiographic examination is necessary and how effectively the radiographic study detects the significant pathology. CT effectively demonstrates the soft tissues and the osseous structures of the canal and provides the important axial view. Already it has replaced many other types of invasive diagnostic procedures, such as myelography, epidural venography, epidurography, and discography, for some problems. Although evaluation of CT is not complete, initial studies have shown that CT demonstrates some pathologic changes, such as a herniated disc, more effectively than the invasive procedures. Furthermore, CT is, of course, a noninvasive study. Although more extensive works on CT of the spine have been published and compendia of papers have been collected, this special volume is obviously very valuable as a summarization of the anatomic information and diagnostic criteria that have been collected by many investigators over the past few years. The objectives of this volume are to provide a practical and integrated manual for the radiologist or clinician interested in CT of the spine, to provide a handbook for performing CT, interpreting images, and selecting patients for scans, and to indicate the present role of CT and conventional radiographic studies of the spine. Although the issue is not all inclusive, the major topics of degenerative diseases, trauma, congenital abnormalities, anatomy, and techniques are covered adequately and succinctly. No more up-to-date coverage is available. The review of spinal tumor pathology as seen by high-resolution CT techniques is the most comprehensive yet published. The chapter on fractures in trauma is detailed and comprehensive. The section on intervertebral discs reviews the previously published and some unpublished CT observations. The chapter contributed by a neurosurgeon illustrates how the CT scan aids in the diagnosis of conditions such as spinal stenosis and in planning and executing surgery.

Victor M. Haughton, M.D.

Contents

Computed Tomography of the Spine

1 Anatomy of the Spine

VICTOR M. HAUGHTON
ALAN L. WILLIAMS

The spinal column and all its associated neural, vascular, and ligamentous structures can be demonstrated with a suitably equipped CT scanner operated with appropriate techniques.[8]

TECHNIQUE

In order to study the spine effectively, a CT scanner must have a tilting gantry with a large aperture. To minimize movement during and between scans, patients are positioned supine and instructed that while x-rays are being generated they should not move, breathe, or, in cervical studies, swallow. Maximal radiation flux and minimal pixel size are chosen to optimize contrast and spatial resolution.[3] A lateral localizer image (digital radiograph) is obtained initially to select optimal gantry angles and slice locations. Contrast enhancement is not used routinely. Reconstructions for sagittal or coronal projections are sometimes useful.

SPINAL CORD

The normal adult spinal cord extends from the cranio-cervical junction to the lower L1 level. With a density between 30 and 40 HU, the cord is easily distinguished from CSF by CT, provided the surrounding subarachnoid space is sufficiently large. When the space is narrower than 2 mm because of an intradural or extradural mass or a congenitally small dural sac, use of intrathecal metrizamide may be necessary to distinguish the cord (Fig. 1.1).

The cord is easily demonstrated in the cervical region.[7, 11] It appears as an oval structure that with present CT techniques has a homogeneous density. The dimensions of the spinal cord in the cervical, thoracic, and upper lumbar regions have been recorded.[5, 11] The cervical enlargement (C5–T1) and thoracic enlargement (T11–L1) represent the portions of the cord that supply the

1

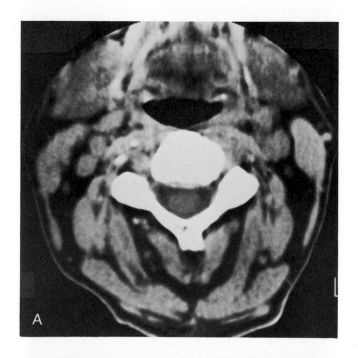

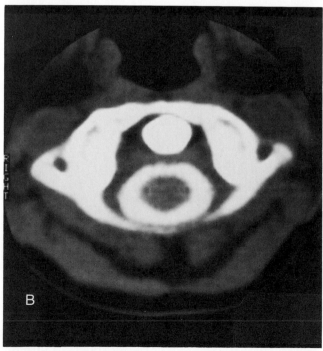

FIG. 1.1 Upper cervical cord. (A) The capacious subarachnoid space at C1 permits excellent visualization of the spinal cord (arrow) without intrathecal contrast medium. (B) Normal spinal cord at C1 in another patient demonstrated with intrathecal metrizamide.

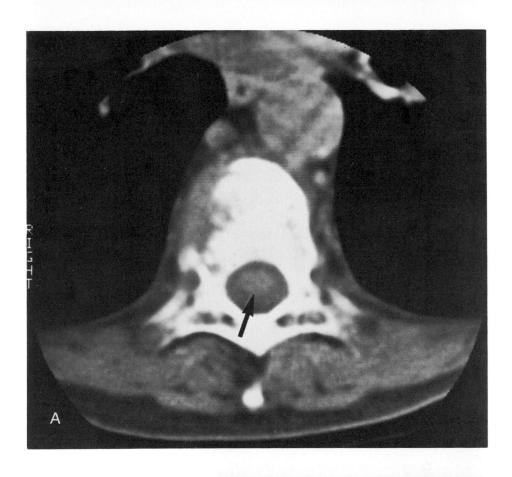

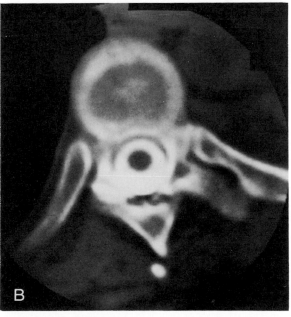

FIG. 1.2 Thoracic cord. (A) When the subarachnoid space is relatively large the spinal cord (arrow) may be demonstrated adequately without intrathecal contrast, as in this patient with metastatic breast carcinoma. (B) Thoracic spinal cord demonstrated by intrathecal contrast.

upper and lower extremities, respectively. When intrathecal contrast is present, the measurement of the cord by CT is affected by window level setting.[10] The most accurate cord measurements result from a window level equidistant between the CT density of the cord and the metrizamide. Because of noise from cardiac motion, and the sometimes small thoracic subarachnoid space, the cord is demonstrated in about two-thirds of thoracic CT studies (Fig. 1.2).[11]

DURAL SAC AND SUBARACHNOID SPACE

A membrane composed of dura and arachnoid encloses the subarachnoid space from the cranio-cervical junction to the second sacral vertebral body. The dural sac is anchored to the coccyx by a filum. Between the dura and the arachnoid is the narrow subdural space. The meninges, having a greater density than cerebrospinal fluid within or surrounding the epidural fat, can be demonstrated in CT, especially if enhanced by an intravenous fusion of iodinated contrast medium.[7, 8] The normal dural sac is round, smooth, and symmetrical (Fig. 1.3). The size of the dural sac is variable and inversely proportional to the amount of epidural fat.

EPIDURAL SPACE

The size and contents of the epidural space varies from region to region. The cervical epidural space is narrow and contains predominantly vascular tissue. In the lumbar region, especially where the caudal dural sac tapers, the epidural space is large and contains substantial amounts of fat. Epidural fat in the thoracic regions varies from patient to patient.[11] Slices at the intervertebral space show more fat than images through the pedicles. Because of its low density, the epidural fat contrasts with the dural sac, axillary pouches, nerves, and veins that it surrounds.

NERVE ROOTS, GANGLIA, AND NERVES

Thirty-one pairs of nerves exit from the vertebral canal to the body. Except for C1 and C2 the nerves exit through the superior aspect of the neural foramen just anterior to the zygoapophyseal (facet) joint. The spinal nerves have motor and sensory roots that arise from the anterior and posterior aspects of the cord, respectively. The posterior dorsal root is larger than the anterior or ventral root and has an enlargement, the gaglion, immediately below the pedicle. The distal portion of each nerve root is surrounded by a sleeve of dura and arachnoid. The nerve roots, nerves, and sheaths vary in size from region to region, with the largest being in the sacral and lower lumbar regions (Fig. 1.4). The cervical (Fig. 1.5) and thoracic nerve roots have a lateral and slightly anterior course; the lumbar nerve roots have a more cephalo-caudad course between the conus and the neural foramen.

The spinal nerves are demonstrated by computed tomography in the paraspinal tissues lateral to the neural foramen (Fig. 1.4C). The root sheaths are noted lateral to the dural sac in the neural foramina (Fig. 1.4A). Nerve roots are demonstrated within the dural sac and root sheaths when intrathecal

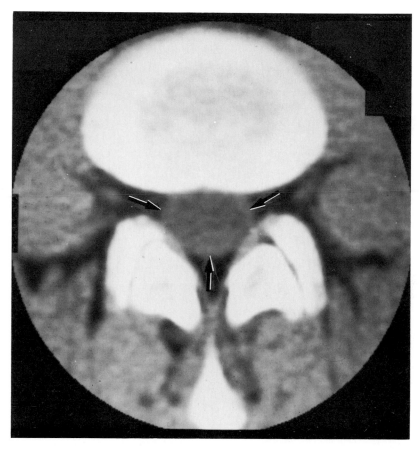

FIG. 1.3 Lumbar dural sac. The normal lumbar dural sac (arrows) is round, smooth, and symmetrical. Epidural fat defines the margins of the dural sac.

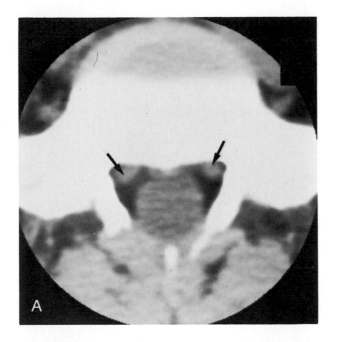

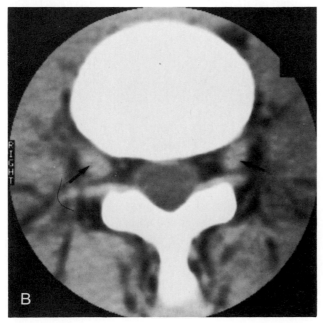

FIG. 1.4 Lumbar root sheaths. (A) Just after the root sheaths separate from the dural sac, they are distinguished in the epidural fat just medial to the pedicle (L5–S1). (B) A cut just inferior to the pedicles shows the ganglia (arrows) in the intervertebral foramina. They are broader than the nerve roots or nerves (L4–L5).

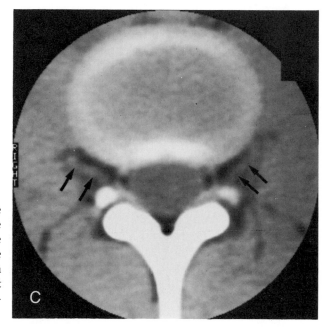

FIG. 1.4 (cont.) (C) The spinal nerves lateral to the intervertebral foramina are demonstrated at a slice through the lowest portion of the neural foramen, at the level of the disc (L4–L5).

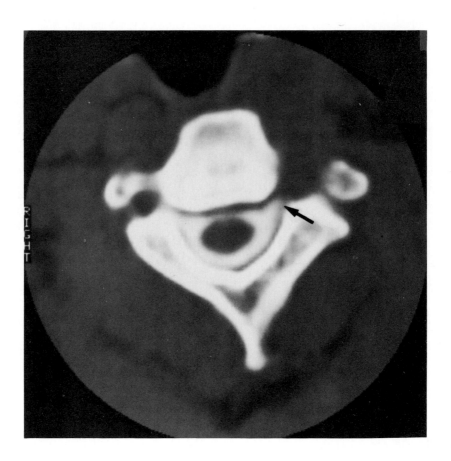

FIG. 1.5   A cervical root sheath (arrow) demonstrated by metrizamide.

metrizamide is used with CT. The cervical nerve root sheaths, oriented in the plane of axial sections, appear rectilinear or triangular in axial CT sections, and can often be traced from the dural sac to the neural foramen (Fig. 1.5); the lumbar nerve roots, perpendicular to an axial CT slice, appear round. An enlargment of the lumbar root sheaths marks the location of the posterior nerve root ganglion (Fig. 1.4B). The portion of the root sheath lateral to the ganglion does not opacify if intrathecal contrast medium is used.

VEINS

In the cervical spine, a venous plexus nearly fills the small epidural space. Therefore, CT resolves no individual cervical epidural veins, but does demonstrate a rim of soft tissue that surrounds (and in CT images blends with) the dural sac and enhances with intravenous contrast medium. In the lumbar region, the epidural veins are surrounded by epidural fat, which makes some of the individual veins discernible in CT. The intraspinal veins consist of the retrovertebral plexus, internal vertebral, basivertebral, transvertebral (or radicular), and epivertebral veins, all of which are interconnected.[8, 9] The anterior internal vertebral veins run longitudinally in the epidural fat anterior and lateral to the dural sac (Fig. 1.6A). Smaller epidural veins are located posterior to the dural sac. The lumbar veins larger than 2 mm in diameter are the ones identified most frequently. The anterior internal vertebral veins may be distinguished from the root sheaths by their smaller size and more medial location. Transvertebral or radicular veins may be identified within the neural foramina (Fig. 1.6B). The veins have a more lateral and horizontal course than the nerve roots and they enhance with contrast medium injected in the ascending lumbar veins. Behind each vertebral body is a retrovertebral plexus (Fig. 1.6C,D). The retrovertebral plexus is denser than the epidural fat, and enhances when contrast medium is injected via ascending lumbar vein catheters. The large retrovertebral plexuses in the lumbar region are often demonstrated by CT. The plexus at each level is connected to the one at the next level by the anterior internal vertebral veins. The basivertebral veins run through the spongiosa of the vertebral bodies to connect the retrovertebral plexus and the epivertebral veins. The Y-shaped channel for the basivertebral vein is usually evident on CT scans in the mid-portion of the vertebral body (Fig. 1.6E,F). A small osseous process may protrude into the vertebral canal at the junction of the retrovertebral plexus and the basivertebral veins. The defect in the vertebra can be distinguished from a destructive process, which it may resemble in some patients, by the small process. This process can be distinguished from an osteophyte by noting its remoteness from the intervertebral disc space.

LIGAMENTS

The ligaments of the vertebral canal demonstrated by CT include the ligamentum flavum, posterior longitudinal, interspinous, and supraspinous ligaments.

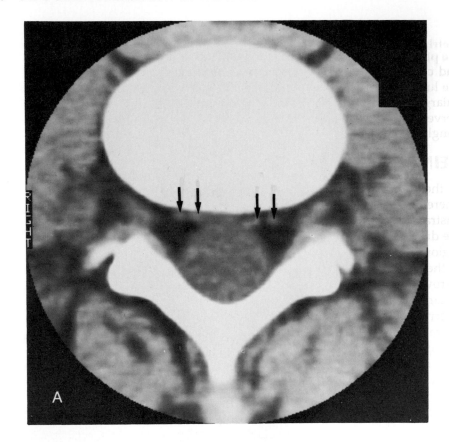

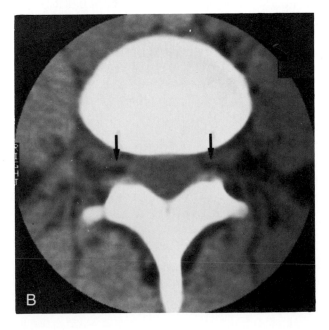

FIG. 1.6 The epidural veins in the lumbar spine. (A) Anterior internal vertebral veins at L4 in cross-section. (B) Transvertebral veins. The transvertebral veins (arrows) within the intervertebral foramina have a more lateral course than the nerves.

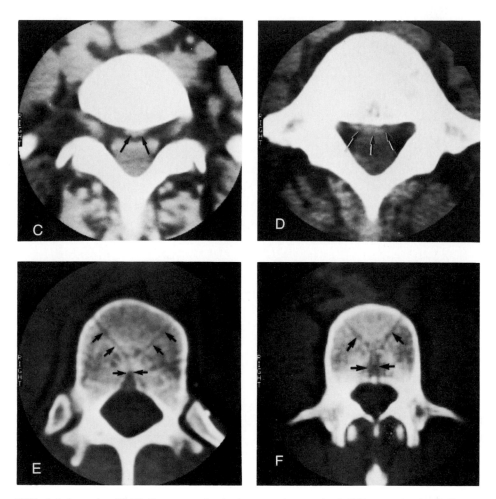

FIG. 1.6 (cont.)   (C,D) Retrovertebral plexuses (arrows) of different size in different patients. (E,F) Basivertebral vein. The Y-shaped channel for the basivertebral vein (arrows) appears similar in both thoracic (E) and lumbar (F) vertebral bodies.

The ligamentum flavum is a thick elastic structure lining the posterolateral aspect of the vertebral canal. Between the atlas and the skull, the ligamentum flavum is a broad, thin membrane (the posterior atlanto-occipital membrane) without a midline split, pierced by the vertebral arteries and C1 nerve roots. The ligament at each vertebral level arises from the anterior surface of the lower edge of one lamina and inserts on the posterior surface of the lamina below. In anatomic sections it is easily recognized because of the yellow color imparted by the elastic fibers. In CT images, the ligamentum flavum has a

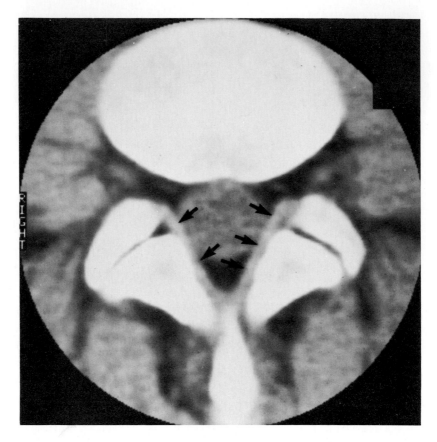

FIG. 1.7   The ligamenta flava (arrows) occupy the posterolateral aspect of the vertebral canal, overlie the facet joint capsule, and extend laterally into the intervertebral foramina.

density intermediate between fat and bone (Fig. 1.7). It appears relatively thin in cuts that include portions of the lamina and relatively thick in cuts that are between laminae. Laterally, the ligamentum flavum blends with the capsule of the facet joints. The average thickness of the normal ligamentum flavum on anatomic sections is 2 to 4 mm.[4]

The posterior longitudinal ligament runs immediately behind the vertebral body. It is incomplete between the occipital bone and C1. In the cervical region it is broad while in the thoracic and lumbar regions it is narrow. It adheres tightly to each annulus fibrosus but is separated from the mid-portion of each vertebral body by vascular and connective tissue. The posterior longitudinal ligament may be recognized in some CT images posterior to the retrovertebral plexus and 3 or 4 mm posterior to the vertebral body (Fig. 1.8).

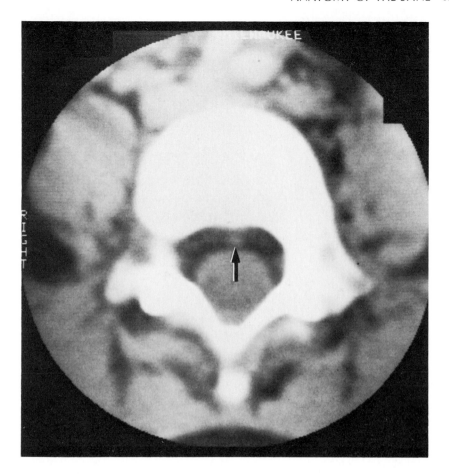

FIG. 1.8 The posterior longitudinal ligament (arrow) can be demonstrated by CT at the level of the vertebral body, where it is separated from the bone by loose connective tissue, but not at the level of the annulus.

The interspinous and supraspinous ligaments may extend the entire length of the spinal canal but may be defective or lacking at some levels. The interspinous ligament between each spinous process is a fibrous connection that is denser than the adjacent connective tissue (Fig. 1.9). The supraspinous ligament begins at the membranous ligamentum nuchae between the occiput and C2 and continues caudally on the tips of the spinous processes.

INTERVERTEBRAL DISC

The intervertebral disc is composed of the central nucleus pulposus, peripheral annulus fibrosus, and cartilaginous vertebral endplate. The annulus contains dense fibrocartilaginous tissue with laminar fibers binding to the ad-

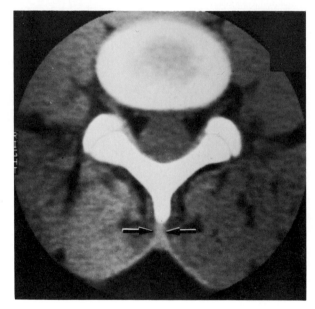

FIG. 1.9 Interspinous ligament. The interspinous ligament (arrows), extending between adjacent spinous processes, is often demonstrated on axial sections.

jacent vertebral endplates. The most peripheral layers contain collaginous fibers that insert in the ring apophysis. The nucleus contains an amorphous, gelatinous material that becomes progressively more fibrotic with age. The cross-sectional shape of the disc conforms to the adjacent vertebral bodies (Figs. 1.10,–1.13). The disc varies in height from 5 to 10 mm in the cervical and thoracic region to 10 to 15 mm in the lumbar.

In CT images, the disc appears homogeneous except at the periphery, which has a greater density because of the collagenous fibers and partial volume artifact associated with the adjacent ring apophysis.

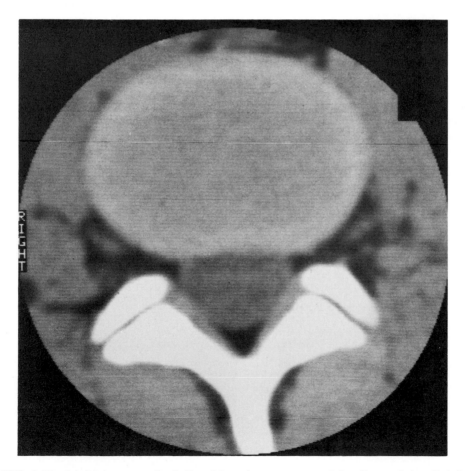

FIG. 1.10 L4–L5 intervertebral disc. Note the symmetry of the disc and the slightly concave posterior margin. The disc is slightly denser than the dural sac and its contents.

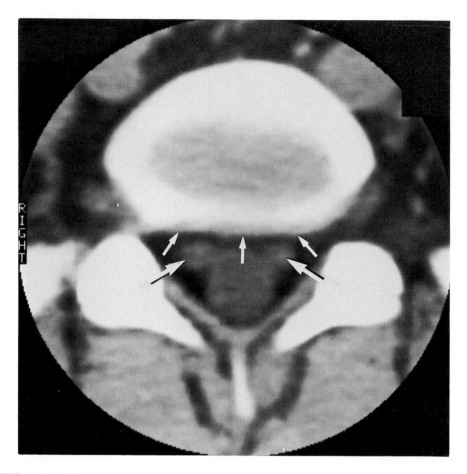

FIG. 1.11   The L5–S1 intervertebral disc has a relatively flat posterior margin (small arrows). The S1 root sheaths (large arrows) are usually identified at the level of the L5–S1 disc.

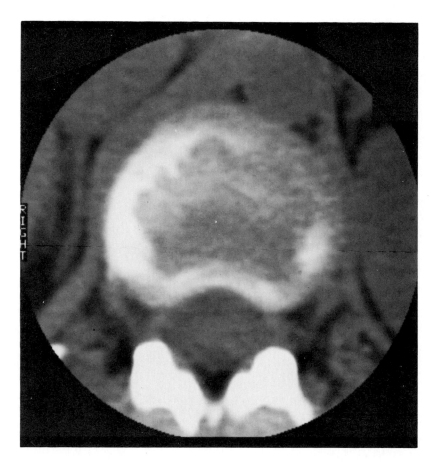

FIG. 1.12   Thoracic intervertebral disc. The normal thoracic disc is concave posteriorly. The greater density in the peripheral disc is the result of partial volume averaging of adjacent osseous endplate.

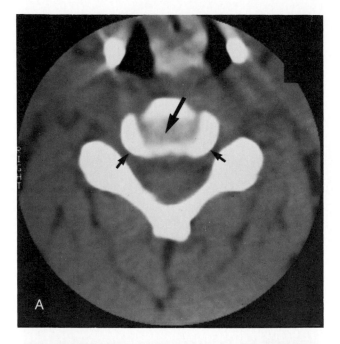

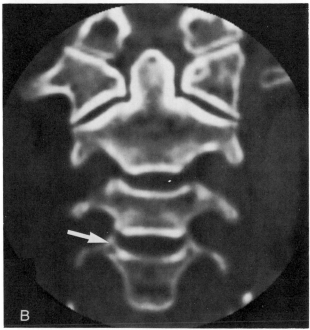

FIG. 1.13 C4–C5 intervertebral disc and uncovertebral joints. The uncinate processes (small arrows) buttress the disc (large arrow) posteriorly. (B) A coronal CT image demonstrates the uncinate process (arrow) forming one side of the uncovertebral joint and intervertebral disc space.

VERTEBRA

The CT appearance of the osseous spine is described in detail elsewhere.[8]

Cervical Vertebrae

The first cervical vertebra has an anterior and posterior arch and lateral masses but no body (Fig. 1.14). The second cervical vertebra is distinctive because of the odontoid process, which articulates with the anterior arch of C1. The vertebral bodies of C3 through C7 are oval in axial projection and broader in transverse than sagittal dimension. The pedicles are oriented posterolaterally.

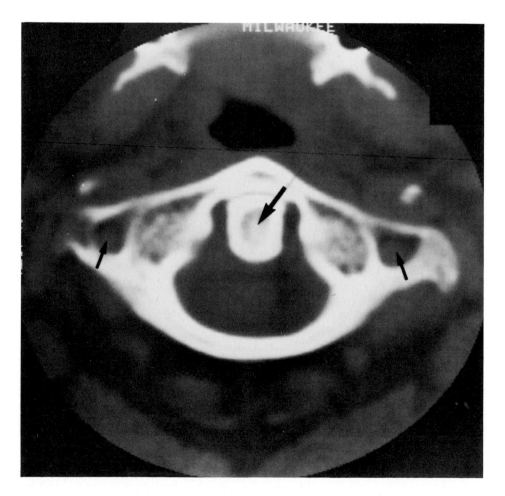

FIG. 1.14   C1 vertebra. The anterior arch articulates with the dens (large arrow). The vertebral arteries (small arrows) pass through the foramina transversaria.

Foramina transversaria containing the vertebral arteries and some veins and sympathetic nerves are located within the transverse processes of C1 through C6, and if the vertebral arteries are aberrant, C7.[11, 13] The spinous processes of C2 and C7, where cervical ligaments and muscles insert, are more prominent than the other spinous cervical processes. The uncinate processes that project superiorly from the lateral margin of the third through seventh cervical vertebra are separated from the adjacent vertebra by the uncovertebral joint, which seldom has a synovial lining and more often contains loose connective tissue, often with a small cleft (Fig. 1.13).[1, 4] The cervical spinal canal changes in configuration from round at C1 and C2 to triangular at C6 and C7.

Thoracic Vertebrae

The thoracic vertebrae are larger than the cervical, more convex anteriorly, and slightly more concave posteriorly. The upper thoracic vertebral bodies have facets for articulation with rib heads. The T10, T11, and T12 vertebrae have short transverse processes that do not articulate with the rib tubercles. The thoracic vertebral pedicles are heavier than the cervical ones and oriented more anteroposteriorly; the thoracic laminae are broader and thicker than the cervical ones and overlap the laminae immediately below. The spinous processes are long and slender and oriented obliquely downward. The thoracic spinal canal is diamond shaped or round in the mid-thoracic region and triangular at either end.

Lumbar Vertebrae

The lumbar vertebral bodies are convex anteriorly, slightly concave posteriorly, and greater in transverse than sagittal diameter. The short, heavy pedicles are oriented anteroposteriorly. The lamina and spinous processes are thick and broad. The size and shape of the lumbar transverse processes vary, particularly that of L5. The fifth lumbar vertebra is particularly subject to developmental anomalies affecting the neural arch, such as spina bifida. The spinal canal at this level is triangular.

Zygoapophyseal (Facet) Joints

The articular processes of adjacent vertebral arches of C3 through S1 articulate by means of synovial, zygoapophyseal, or facet joints. The paired facet joints are usually symmetrical. The normal thickness of opposing articular process cartilage and joint space is 2 to 4 mm (Fig. 1.15).[2] The facet joints are supplied by recurrent branches from the posterior primary rami of the spinal nerves. The cortical margins are uniformly thick, and straight or slightly curving. The plane of the facet joints varies from region to region. The vertically oriented facet joints of the lumbar region are very effectively demonstrated and studied by CT.

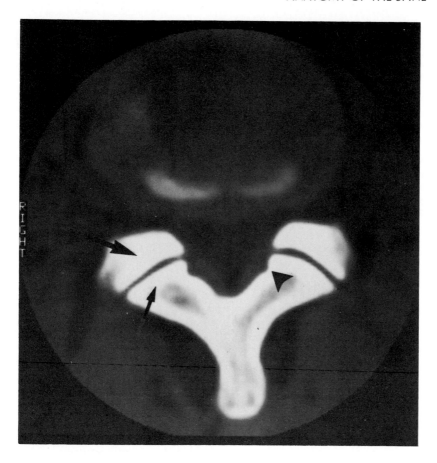

FIG. 1.15 Zygoapophyseal (facet) joints. The superior (large arrow) and inferior (small arrow) articular processes are symmetrical. These synovial joints are located at the level of the intervertebral disc. Note the notch where the synovium attaches to the inferior articular process (arrowhead).

References

1. Boreadis AG, Gershon-Cohen J: Luschka joints of the cervical spine. Radiology 66:181–187, 1956.
2. Carrera GF, Haughton VM, Syvertsen A, Williams AL: Computed tomography of the lumbar facet joints. Radiology 134:145–148, 1980.
3. Cohen G: Contrast-detail-dose analysis of six different computed tomographic scanners. J Comput Assist Tomogr 3:197–203, 1979.
4. Ebstein BS: The Spine—A Radiological Text and Atlas (4th ed.). pp. 24–83. Lea & Febiger, Philadelphia, 1976.
5. Elliott HC: Cross-sectional diameters and areas of human spinal cord. Anat Res 93:287–293, 1945.

6. Glenn WV, Rhodes ML, Altschuler EM, Wilse LL, Kostanek C, Kuo YM: Multiplanar display computerized body tomography applications in the lumbar spine. Spine 4:202–352, 1979.

7. Haughton VM, Syvertsen A, Williams AL: Soft tissue anatomy within the spinal canal as seen on CT. Radiology 134:649–656, 1980.

8. Haughton VM, Williams AL: Computed Tomography of the Spine, CV Mosby, St. Louis, 1982.

9. Parke WW: Applied Anatomy of the Spine. In Rothman RH and Simeone FA, Eds.: The Spine. WB Saunders, Philadelphia, 1975.

10. Seibert CE, Barnes JE, Dreisbach JN, Swanson WI, Heck RJ: Accurate CT measurement of the spinal cord using metrizamide: Physical factors. AJR 136:777–780, 1981.

11. Taylor AJ, Haughton VM, Doust BD: CT imaging of the thoracic spinal cord without intrathecal contrast medium. J Comput Assist Tomogr 4:223–224, 1980.

2 Intervertebral Disc Degeneration

VICTOR M. HAUGHTON

The excellent images that CT provides of the intervertebral disc suggested its application to diagnosis of disc herniation.[1] Logically, an axial image that shows the entire peripheral margin of the disc at once should demonstrate a herniation more effectively than a coronal or even a sagittal image. Furthermore, a direct image of the disc should demonstrate herniations more accurately than an indirect investigation of disc pathology such as myelography or venography. To date, none of the radiographic modalities available for studying the intervertebral disc have provided the accuracy desired. Therefore, as soon as high-resolution CT scanners were available, they were evaluated for the diagnosis of herniated intervertebral discs.[2, 3] These evaluations already justify the use of CT as the primary diagnostic modality for studying the intervertebral discs and as the sole modality in the majority of cases.[4]

The purpose of this chapter is to review the CT appearance of degenerated intervertebral discs. For the purposes of discussion, disc disease can be divided into bulging of the annulus and herniation of the nucleus pulposus. Because they present somewhat different clinical or radiographic problems, for discussion herniations can be divided into lateral, far-lateral, central, and extruded fragments. The differential diagnosis of disc herniations will introduce a few other types of spinal anomalies or pathology.

TECHNIQUES

For spinal imaging, the patient should be positioned supine, informed about the procedure, and instructed to hold his breath during the imaging process and to lie as quietly as possible. For cervical imaging, the patient should also be instructed not to swallow. In some scanners, additional absorbing material should be placed around the neck.[5]

With axial images through the intervertebral disc excluding the adjacent vertebral end-plates, CT diagnosis of herniated disc is very effective. To obtain these axial images, a localizer image is used to locate the plane and level of each intervertebral disc space of interest (Fig. 2.1). In addition to the cut within the plane of the disc, sufficient contiguous cuts are obtained above and below to encompass the adjacent neural foramina. In the lumbar region, a series of five contiguous 5-mm-thick slices with the central slice centered on the intervertebral disc is usually satisfactory; in the cervical region, a series of five or seven cuts 1.5 mm thick are usually required. Since contrast and spatial resolution are critical for the CT study of the spine, techniques should be chosen to minimize pixel size and maximize the radiation flux. Therefore, we

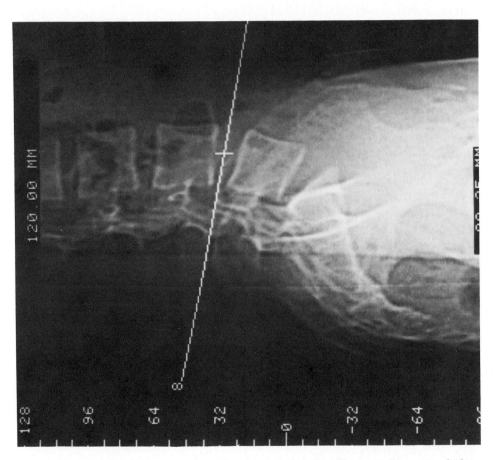

FIG. 2.1   A lateral localizer image with a cursor placed to illustrate the optimal plane for imaging the L4–L5 intervertebral disc. An axial section 5 mm thick in this plane and four contiguous cuts (two above and two below) are required to study the disc and the neural foramina at this level. For the L5–S1 disc, a slightly different gantry angle and a second series of five cuts will be needed.

use 500 to 600 Ma., 1150 Ma.S., and either small calibration or (especially in very obese patients or near the shoulder region) large calibration and target reconstruction.

An alternative technique is to obtain contiguous or overlapping slices with a vertical gantry. This technique may be preferable when an adequate localizer scan is not available or the unusual situation when a reformatted sagittal or coronal image is anticipated. The disadvantage of the technique is that images made in planes not perpendicular to the rostro-caudal axis of the spine have geometric distortion and partial volume average errors. As a result of these, the dimensions of the spinal canal and neural foramina may be underestimated and disc margins may be less reliably resolved. Some authors have advocated the combination of the two techniques, which increases the radiation exposure without improving the accuracy of the study substantially.

Contrast enhancement technique has little application in the study of intervertebral disc disease. Contrast enhancement with approximately 40 g (as iodine) of intravenous contrast medium may be useful in some cases to distinguish a scar, which increases in density after enhancement, from a herniated disc fragment, which theoretically does not. Intrathecal contrast enhancement can be performed by injecting approximately 5 g (as iodine) of metrizamide into the subarachnoid space, tilting the patient to move the contrast medium into the region of interest and then CT imaging. Intrathecal enhancement seldom facilitates diagnosis of herniated disc and in fact may degrade the image of the epidural space but helps to identify a conjoint root sheath, which simulates a herniated disc.

BULGING ANNULUS

Degeneration of the intervertebral discs causes shrinkage of the nucleus pulposus and laxity of the fibers in the annulus fibrosis. As a result, the inner layers of the annulus bulge centripetally and the outer layers bulge centrifugally. The net result is a disc with cross-sectional area larger than that of the normal disc or adjacent vertebrae. Bulging discs commonly narrow the spinal canal, compress the dural sac, and often constrict the inferior portion of the neural foramen, but seldom compress the spinal nerves that are located in the upper portion of the neural foramina. Therefore, the bulging disc rarely produces radiculopathy.

Computed tomography shows the margins of a bulging disc extending beyond the adjacent vertebral bodies (Fig. 2.2).[6] The entire disc circumference is abnormal, usually symmetrically, except in scoliosis. The posterior margin of a bulging disc may retain its normal concavity or become convex. CT usually shows a cushion of fat separating the bulging disc margin from the spinal nerve in the neural foramen. If CT shows all the fat in the neural foramen obliterated in a patient with sciatica, nerve compression can be suspected. Often CT shows gas replacing portions of the nucleus pulposus (vacuum disc phenomenon) in a bulging annulus.

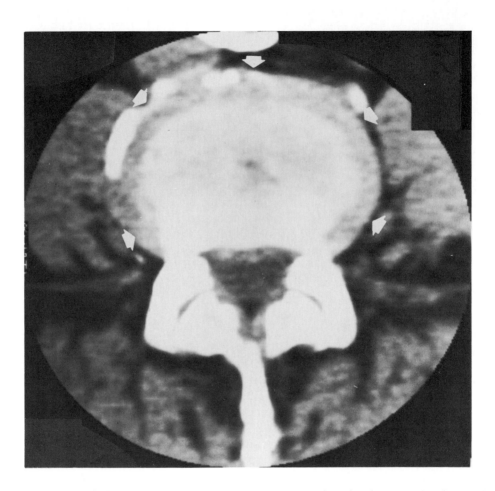

FIG. 2.2 A bulging disc demonstrated by CT. Note that the disc margins (arrows) extend beyond the adjacent vertebra.

HERNIATED DISC

In the degenerative process, some fibers in the annulus fibrosis weaken and tear. If all layers of the annulus tear, the nucleus pulposus herniates from its normal position to a location outside the annulus. The most common location for the tears, either because of intrinsic weakness of the fibers or their greater curvature, is the posterolateral regions of the disc. The posterior longitudinal ligament that reinforces the annulus fibrosis, especially in the midline, may prevent the herniated fragment from escaping free into the spinal canal or neural foramen but not from its compressing a spinal nerve.

A disc herniation confined behind the posterior longitudinal ligament appears in CT images as a focally protruding disc margin with a smooth curvilinear margin (Fig. 2.3).[3] The density of the herniated nucleus pulposus and the remainder of the disc are usually the same. The herniated disc displaces epidural fat, often compresses the dural sac, and stretches a nerve or root sheath in the spinal canal or the neural foramen. A normal sheath has epidural fat completely surrounding it, an affected one does not. Therefore, the displaced nerve may be obscured by the herniated nuclear fragment. The obscuring of a nerve root by a herniated disc is an important sign. Unless nerve root compression can be identified by CT, radicular signs probably should not be attributed to the disc herniation.

If the nuclear herniation penetrates the posterior longitudinal ligament as well as the annulus, the nuclear fragment is called free or extruded. If the fragment lies adjacent to the posterior disc margin, the disc margin will be abnormal, usually with a polypoid configuration rather than the smooth, curvilinear one of the subligamentous herniation. Some cases of a free fragment in a lateral recess or within the spinal canal are obvious (Fig. 2.4). If a free fragment lies in the posterior part of the spinal canal and not contiguous with the disc margin, the intervertebral disc margin may appear normal in the CT study. In these cases the fragment may simulate a root sheath or anomalous dural sac. A free fragment having greater density than the dural sac or root sheath can be detected by careful inspection or density measurements (Fig. 2.5). In questionable cases, a metrizamide-enhanced CT study or myelogram may be useful.

Far lateral disc herniations may have different clinical, surgical and myelographic findings than other herniations. Because the nuclear fragment compresses the spinal nerve peripheral to the posterior nerve root ganglion, the mechanical signs detected on physical examination may be atypical. At laminectomy, a routine inspection of the spinal canal without probing into the neural foramen or foramenotomy may be negative. Furthermore, myelography is relatively insensitive for the far lateral disc herniation since the normal root sheath, proximal to the herniation, is visualized during myelography. Therefore, the CT examination is extremely important to identify far lateral disc herniations.[7] CT shows a tissue with the density of disc (80–120 HU) replacing fat in the neural foramen and obscuring of the spinal nerve

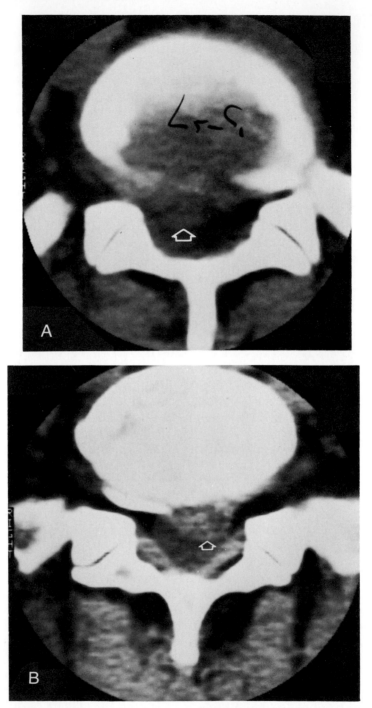

FIG. 2.3 Four examples of subligamentous herniations at L5–S1 demonstrated in CT as a focal smooth protrusion of the disc margin. (A,B) illustrate the smooth border of a subligamentous herniation;

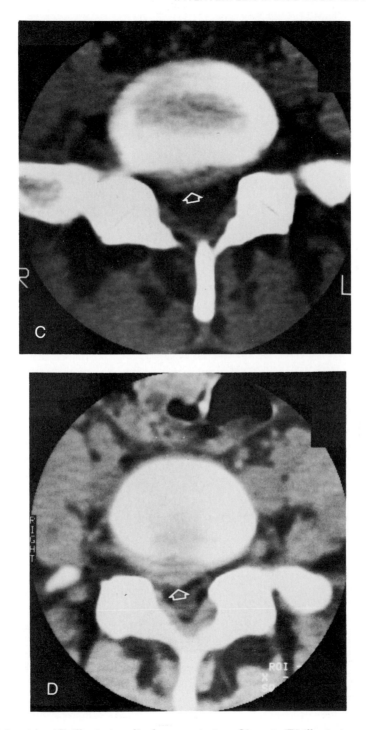

FIG. 2.3 (cont.)   (C) illustrates displacement at an S1 root; (D) illustrates a large herniation with a small dural sac.

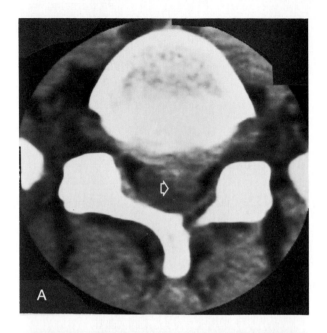

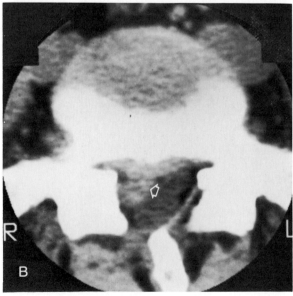

FIG. 2.4 Four examples of extruded disc herniations (free fragments). In (A) the extruded fragment (arrow) is contiguous with a larger subligamentous fragment. In (B) the free fragment (arrow) is separated from the posterior disc margin that is nearly normal.

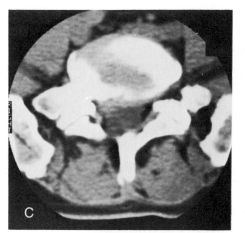
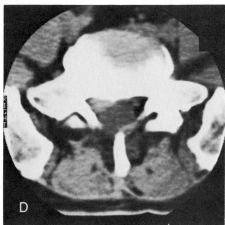
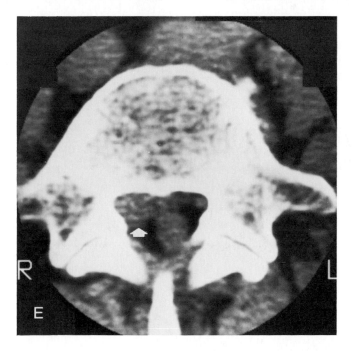

FIG. 2.4 (cont.) (C,D) Contiguous slices through a fragment in the lateral recess. Note that the slice below the disc (D) shows the fragment more effectively than the slice at the disc (C). (E) A free fragment (arrow) that could be mistaken for a large root sheath. However, asymmetry to this degree is unusual for root sheaths and the fragment is denser than the normal sheath.

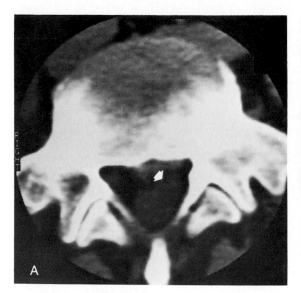

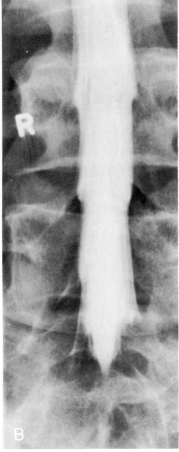

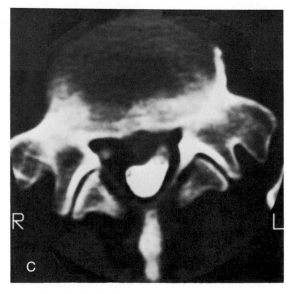

FIG. 2.5 Conjoint root sheaths. The anomalous left S1 root sheath (arrow) resembles the free fragment seen in Figure 2.4E. A herniation is excluded by the myelogram (B) or the CT scan with metrizamide in the subarachnoid space (C).

(Fig. 2.6). A neurofibroma that produces no bony changes in the neural foramen may be difficult to differentiate from a far lateral herniation[10] (see Chapter 4).

Central disc herniations are not infrequent although they are rarely the cause of sciatic symptoms. CT shows them as smooth, curvilinear, midline protrusions of the disc margin, often indenting the dural sac but not compressing a spinal nerve. A central disc herniation demonstrated by CT should not be considered clinically significant unless the clinical findings are explained by a midline process.

ACCURACY OF CT

Several investigators have compared CT with myelography in the diagnosis of herniated disc.[4, 8, 9] High-resolution CT has in each study demonstrated intervertebral disc herniations more reliably than myelography. Specifically, disc herniations at the L5–S1 level (Fig. 2.3D) or far lateral in the neural foramen (Fig. 2.6B,C), or in patients with small dural sacs (Fig. 2.3D) have been more difficult to detect with myelography than with CT. The potential failures of CT are 1) overlooking a conus medullaris tumor that clinically simulates a lower lumbar intervertebral disc herniation; 2) missing a herniated disc at L3–L4 because only the two lower discs are studied;[9] or 3) identifying a herniation when epidural fat is scarce, either because of previous surgery or a narrow spinal canal from a large dural sac.[4] In all studies of CT, anatomic confirmation is a problem. Utilization of surgical results for confirmation may lead to some errors but practically speaking represents the best verification available.

DIFFERENTIAL DIAGNOSIS

In the differential diagnosis of herniated discs, four processes must be considered: conjoint root sheath, spondylolisthesis, epidural tumor, and epidural scar.

In a dural sac anomaly, the pattern of epidural fat may be asymmetric and abnormal. When a root sheath has a broader than normal connection with the dural sac, in, for example, a conjoint root sheath, a herniated disc may be simulated in the axial CT images (Fig. 2.5). However, the conjoint root sheath has a nearly homogeneous density whereas the free fragment has greater density than the dural sac. In scoliosis, an axial CT slice may intersect the root sheaths asymmetrically so that the epidural fat appears deficient on one side. This condition must also be distinguished from a free fragment.

The intervertebral disc is distorted if the vertical alignment is abnormal. In spondylolisthesis, the posterior disc margin extends beyond one of the adjacent vertebrae. At the level of a spondylolisthesis, CT shows posterior disc margin protruding symmetrically beyond the higher vertebral body. Although this protrusion may suggest herniation, it is more symmetrical than the usual herniation and not in contact with one of the spinal nerves (see

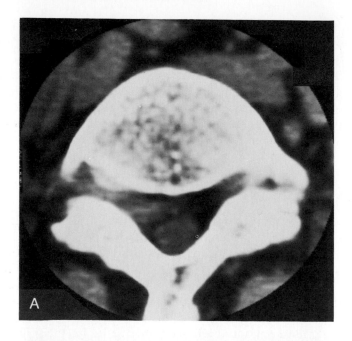

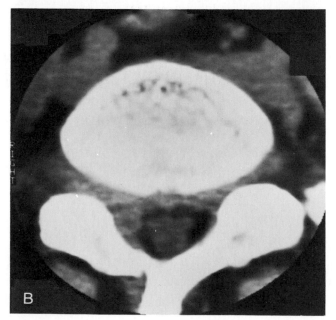

FIG. 2.6 Examples of lateral and far lateral herniated discs. (A,B) Two contiguous cuts in patients with a right sided herniation. On the higher cut (A) the L5 nerve on the right is obscured by the fragment; on (B) the S1 root sheath emerging from the dural sac at this level is separated from the fragment by fat and is therefore unaffected.

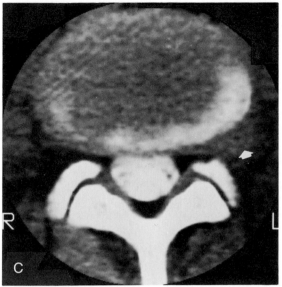

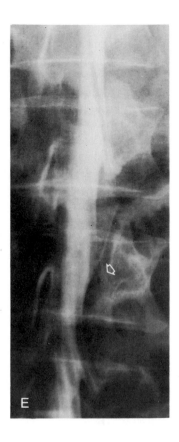

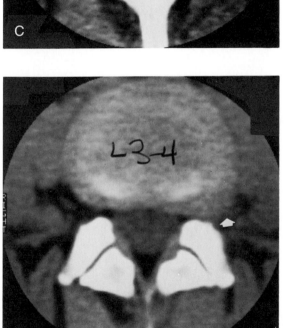

FIG. 2.6 (cont.) (C) Another far lateral herniation (arrow) at L3–L4. (D,E) Myelograms and CT in another patient. The herniation (arrow) is easily seen in the CT scan and causes a subtle change in the myelographic appearance of the L3 root sheath (open arrow).

Chapter 7). When the margin appears asymmetric or compresses the spinal nerve, a disc herniation must be suspected. We have seen several examples of disc herniation in conjunction with spondylolisthesis (Fig. 2.7).

An epidural tumor displacing fat may simulate a herniated disc. Most epidural processes are malignant and, therefore, have bony changes that distinguish them from a herniated disc (see Chapter 4). Careful evaluation of the bone adjacent to a soft-tissue mass is necessary to detect metastases, lymphoma, and myeloma that may alter the epidural space as a herniation does. The benign tumors in the epidural space like neurofibroma usually demonstrate some bony atrophy. However, at least one case of a neurofibroma without bony atrophy has been reported with CT findings very similar to that of a herniated disc.[10]

Epidural scar and recurrent herniated disc may be difficult to distinguish by CT since both are characterized by replacement of epidural fat with a higher-density tissue (Fig. 2.8). Some features may distinguish the two. A scar usually retracts the dural sac whereas a disc herniation displaces it. One investigator uses intravenous contrast enhancement to identify scar tissue and exclude herniated disc on the assumption that a herniation never enhances.[11] Some investigators have criteria for distinguishing scar from her-

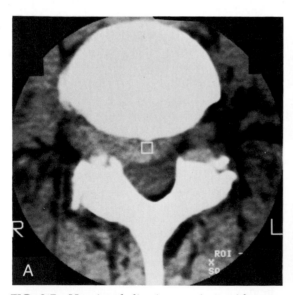

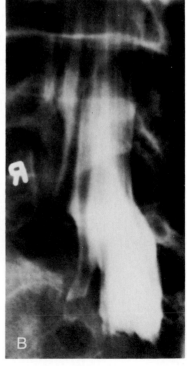

FIG. 2.7 Herniated disc in a patient with spondylolysis. (A) The asymmetric posterior disc margin is typical of herniated disc, not the distortion due to a spondylolisthesis (see Chapter 7). Compression of the right fifth nerve seen in the CT image was confirmed by myelography (B).

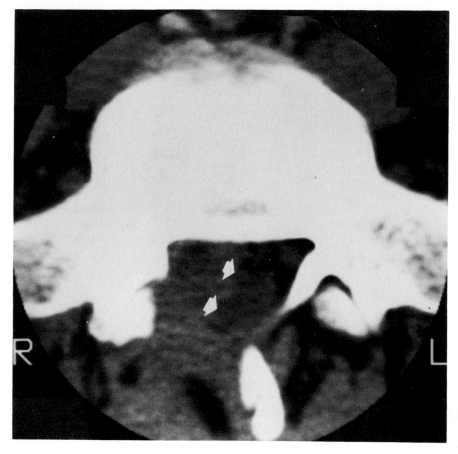

FIG. 2.8   Epidural fibrosis. The dural sac (arrows) is displaced by a large scar secondary to the previous laminectomy and removal of a herniated disc fragment (same patient as 4B).

niated disc with the subarachnoid space enhanced with metrizamide.[12] Density measurements have been used to distinguish scar, which ordinarily has a density under 80 HU, from a disc herniation, which is usually above 80 HU. We have found, however, that one of these criteria are completely reliable. Furthermore, in the postoperative patient, distinguishing scar from herniated disc is not so important as identifying a localized mass of abnormal tissue in the epidural space that correlates precisely with clinical symptomatology. This latter situation has surgical implications if a disc herniation or scar is present. Localized abnormalities that do not correlate with the clinical symptomatology or diffuse abnormalities in the epidural space have less clinical significance.

References

1. Haughton VM, Syvertsen A, Williams AL: Soft-tissue anatomy within the spinal canal as seen on computed tomography. Radiology 134:649–655, 1980.

2. Meyer GA, Haughton VM, Williams AL: Diagnosis of herniated lumbar disk with computed tomography. N Engl J Med 301:1166–1167, 1979.

3. Williams AL, Haughton VM, Syvertsen A: Computed tomography in the diagnosis of herniated nucleus pulposus. Radiology 135:95–99, 1980.

4. Haughton VM, Eldevik OP, Magnaes B, Amundsen P: A prospective comparison of computed tomography and myelography in the diagnosis of herniated lumbar disks. Radiology 142:103–110, 1982.

5. Orrison W, Johansen JG, Eldevik OP, Haughton VM: Optimal computer tomographic techniques for cervical spine imaging. Radiology 144:180–182, 1982.

6. Williams AL, Haughton VM, Meyer GA, Ho KC: Computed tomographic appearance of the bulging annulus. Radiology 142:403–408, 1982.

7. Williams AL, Haughton VM, Daniels DL, Thornton RS: CT recognition of lateral disk herniation. Am J Neuroradiol 3:211–214, 1982.

8. Raskin SP, Keating JW: Recognition of lumbar disk disease: Comparison of myelography and computed tomography. Am J Neuroradiol 3:215–222, 1982.

9. Gado MH, Chandra-Sekar B, Patel J, Hodges FJ, Kapila A: An integrated approach to the diagnosis of lumbar disc disease by computed tomography and myelography. 67th Meeting of the Radiological Society of North America, Chicago, October 16, 1981.

10. Yang WC, Zappulla R, Malis L: Neurolemmoma in lumbar intervertebral foramen. J Comput Assist Tomogr 5:904–906, 1981.

11. Schubiger O, Valavanis A: CT differentiation between recurrent disc herniation and postoperative scar formation: the value of contrast enhancement. Neuroradiology 22:251–254, 1982.

12. Meyer JD, Latchaw RE, Roppolo HM, Ghoshhajra K, Deeb Z: Computed tomography and myelography of the postoperative lumbar spine. Am J Neuroradiol 3:223–228, 1982.

3 Lumbar Facet Arthropathy

GUILLERMO F. CARRERA

INTRODUCTION

Computed tomographic study of large numbers of patients with chronic low back and sciatic pain has revealed a large population of patients with abnormalities of the lumbar facet joints.[1, 2] Intrinsic lumbar facet arthropathy has long been appreciated as a significant cause for low back pain and pain referred to the sciatic distribution.[3-7] Conventional radiographic findings in lumbar facet arthropathy are frequently nonspecific, and myelographic examination does not adequately study the osteoarticular envelope of the lumbar canal. Patients with symptomatic lumbar facet arthropathy, therefore, have generally been identified using clinical criteria supported by negative myelography. Plain films of the spine were primarily used as a screening examination, searching for neoplastic, inflammatory, or traumatic lesions. Prior to the general acceptance of CT as the best technique for evaluating the lumbar spine in cases of mechanical backache, symptomatic lumbar facet arthropathy remained a diagnosis of exclusion and was frequently impossible to discriminate from myofascial syndrome[3, 5, 7] and other conditions, both organic and functional, presenting as backache and sciatica.

High-resolution CT is now recognized as the best way to discriminate patients with herniated disc, spinal canal and neural foraminal deformity, lumbar facet arthritis, and spondylolysis.[1, 2, 8-10] This potential for effective diagnosis has reawakened interest in selectively evaluating patients with CT evidence for lumbar facet arthritis using selective joint injection. In this way patients with symptomatic lumbar facet arthropathy can be accurately diagnosed and in some cases effectively treated.[7, 11, 12]

ANATOMY AND PATHOPHYSIOLOGY

The lumbar facet joints are paired, diarthrodial articulations between the inferior articular facets of a lumbar segment and the superior articular facets of the segment below. The plane of the articular surfaces is oblique to the coronal anatomic plane and the joints are usually curved with the concavity of the joint toward the spinous process. (Fig. 3.1)

The lumbar facet capsule is re-enforced and partially formed by spinal ligamentous structures, and contains a redundant synovium overlying well-developed fat pads that fill the superior and inferior recesses of the joint.[13] Anatomic studies have shown richly innervated synovial-adipose villi extending from the superior and inferior fat pads well into the articular space of the lumbar facet joints in normal individuals.[14] The sensory innervation of the lumbar facet joints is derived from recurrent branches of the posterior primary rami. Each facet joint receives innervation from the posterior primary ramus of the spinal nerve at its own level as well as descending nerve fibers from the level above. (Fig. 3.2).[15, 16] Since each facet joint receives sensory innervation from more than one spinal level, pain originating in any lumbar facet joint can be referred to the distribution of at least two spinal nerve roots. Lumbar facet arthropathy is classically described as causing pain or muscle

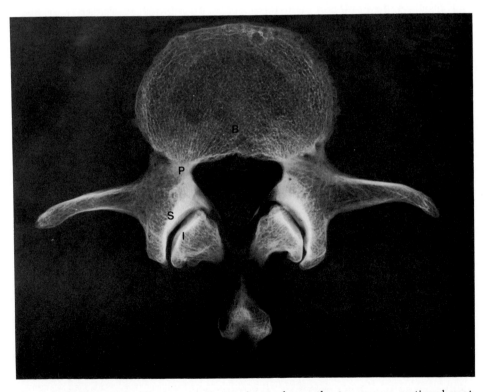

FIG. 3.1 Radiograph of an anatomic specimen shows the transverse sectional anatomy of the L4–L5 lumbar facet joints. B = vertebral body L5; P = right pedicle L5; S = superior articular facet L5; I = inferior articular facet L4 (With permission from Carrera, GF: Lumbar facet joint injection in low back pain and sciatica (I) and II. Radiology 136:661–667, 1980.)

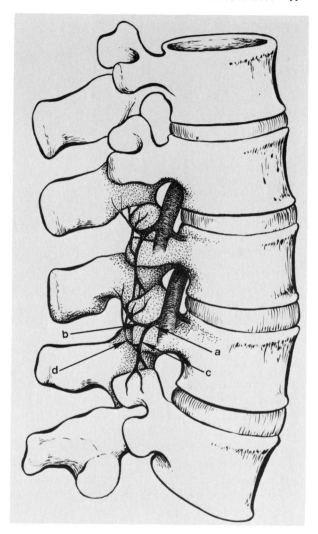

FIG. 3.2 Diagrammatic representation of the innervation of the lumbar facet joints. The posterior primary ramus (a) divides into a lateral branch (b), which supplies the facet joint, capsule, and surrounding soft tissues at its own level, and a medial branch (c), which descends to supply the joint below as well as surrounding tissues. Recurrent fibers from the medial branches (d) ascend to supply the joint at the level of origin of the posterior primary ramus as well.

spasm in the distribution of the spinal sclerotomes, rather than the cutaneous dermatomes, reflecting the sclerotomal origin of the deep osteoarticular structures.[5, 7]

CT OF THE LUMBAR FACET JOINTS

The lumbar facet joints lie at, or near the transaxial level of the intervertebral discs. They are effectively studied using the same images obtained for evaluating the spinal canal in suspected herniated disc. Numerous protocols have been proposed for efficient evaluation of the lumbar spine.[17] We prefer to perform contiguous, 5-mm slices in the plane of the intervertebral disc as determined by preliminary lateral localizer image (ScoutView®). (Fig. 3.3) Five or six contiguous cuts, one in the plane of the disc, and two or three on either

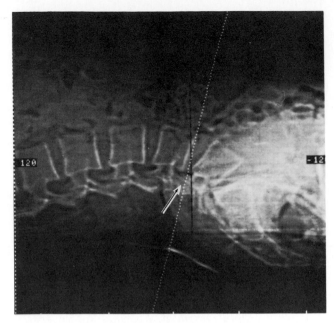

FIG. 3.3 Lateral localizer (Scoutview®) image shows the cursors at the level (dark line) and gantry angle (dotted line) for transverse imaging of the L4–L5 intervertebral disc and L4–L5 facet Joints (arrow). (With permission from Carrera, GF et al.: Computed tomography of the lumbar facet joints. Radiology 134:145, 1980.)

side, are usually sufficient for studying the region of the intervertebral disc, neural formina, and pars interarticularis. Additional cuts may occasionally be necessary. For maximum resolution of the soft-tissue structures, a 10-sec scan time, 25 cm ("infant calibration") field of view, 120 Kv and 960–1152 mA are routinely employed. These factors provide contrast resolution less than 0.5 percent, spatial resolution 0.75mm and radiation dose of 4 rads per examination to the skin. The lumbar facet joints are studied using image windows appropriate for demonstrating bone detail (window width 1000–4000 HU and level of 250–350 HU).

Normal lumbar facet joints show parallel, smooth subchondral bone with a clear demarcation between the subarticular cortex and the medullary space. Normal facet joints measure between 2.0 and 4.0 mm, and are variably curved. (Fig. 3.4)

One of the most frequent finding in patients with abnormal lumbar facet joints is hypertrophy of one of the articular facets. Most commonly the superior articular facet is noted to enlarge, with preservation of the corticomedullary discrimination. (Fig. 3.5) Osteophytes, a common finding in degenerative arthritis of the radicular skeleton are also a frequent abnormality in patients with lumbar facet disease. Osteophytes, in contrast to simple hypertrophy of an articular facet, are uniformly dense structures that project beyond normal cortical boundaries at the articular margins. (Fig. 3.6)

Joint narrowing, reactive subchondral sclerosis, and articular erosions are common abnormalities in primary and secondary degenerative arthritis. These abnormalities are easily demonstrated on CT images of the lumbar facet

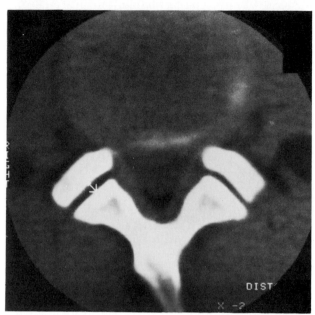

FIG. 3.4 CT image through normal L4–L5 facet joints, which are relatively straight (in contrast to those shown in Figure 3.1). Computer program has been used to measure the right joint to be 0.3 cm wide. (With permission from Carrera, GF et al.: Computed tomography of the lumbar facet joints. Radiology 134:145, 1980.)

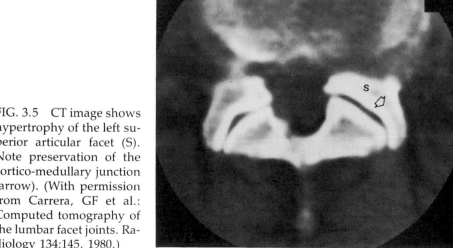

FIG. 3.5 CT image shows hypertrophy of the left superior articular facet (S). Note preservation of the cortico-medullary junction (arrow). (With permission from Carrera, GF et al.: Computed tomography of the lumbar facet joints. Radiology 134:145, 1980.)

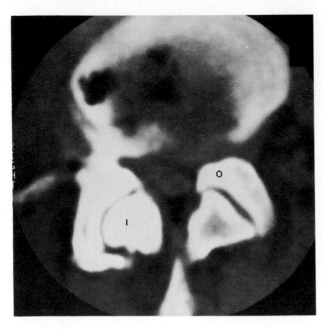

FIG. 3.6 CT image through the L5–S1 facet joints show severe degenerative changes. Large osteophytes (O) project anteriorly from the left superior articular facet of S1, and posteriorly from the right superior facet of S1. The right joint is severely narrowed, and there is marked sclerosis of the right inferior facet of L5 (I). (With permission from Carrera, GF et al.: Computed tomography of the lumbar facet joints. Radiology, 134:145, 1980.)

joints. (Fig. 3.6, 3.7) Subchondral erosions are relatively uncommon in the lumbar facet joints, but imply severe arthritis with considerable destruction of subchondral bone.

Calcification of the lumbar facet capsule is a surprisingly frequent CT finding in patients with abnormal lumbar facet joints. (Fig. 3.8) Conventional radiography demonstrates this finding very rarely in the radicular skeleton in patients without a disorder of calcium metabolism or crystal deposition. It is possible that the improved contrast resolution possible with CT demonstrates calcification in articular capsules that would not be demonstrated by conventional radiographic techniques.

CT scanning can effectively identify a substantial population of patients with lumbar facet arthropathy among those being studied for backache and sciatica. (Table 3.1) The information provided by CT, however, is anatomic only, and cannot discriminate patients whose symptoms are originating in the facet joints. Since CT can accomplish the important step of finding patients at risk for symptomatic facet arthropathy, however, it is therefore possible to selectively apply intra-articular injection to identify patients with symptomatic lumbar facet arthropathy.

LUMBAR FACET INJECTION

Intra-articular lumbar facet block using local anesthetics and cortico-steroid suspensions has been applied to the diagnosis and treatment of patients with symptomatic lumbar facet arthropathy.[7, 11] Patients who meet the clinical criteria for lumbar facet syndrome, and who have CT evidence of lumbar facet arthropathy should be evaluated using fluoroscopically guided lumbar facet block.

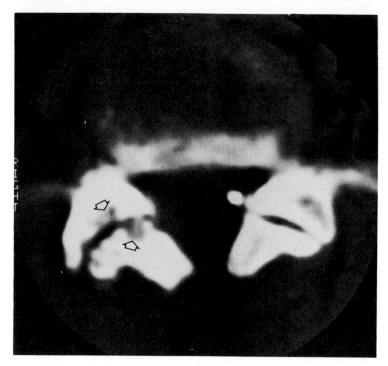

FIG. 3.7 CT image through the L5–S1 facet joints in a postoperative patient. Extensive degenerative changes including severe subchondral sclerosis and erosions (arrows) are evident in the right joint. A drop of residual myelographic contrast is adjacent to the less diseased left joint. (With permission from Carrera, GF et al.: Computed tomography of the lumbar facet joints. Radiology 134:145, 1980.)

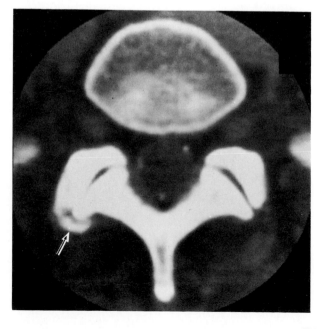

FIG. 3.8 CT through the L5–S1 facet joints shows curved calcification of the posterior joint capsule on the right (arrow).

TABLE 3.1 CT findings in 1000 patients studied for sciatica

Total patients studied	1000
Lumbar facet arthropathy	432
Herniated disc	181

Lumbar facet joint injection is accomplished following direct puncture of the lumbar facet joints using fluoroscopic control. Abnormal joints at levels that could account for the patient's symptoms, as shown by CT, are appropriately selected for blocking. It is rarely necessary to inject more than two joints, and only one side should need blocking in most cases. If a patient with bilateral radiating pain is examined, only one side should be blocked initially to confirm the diagnosis of facet syndrome.

After the lumbar facet joint is visualized fluoroscopically with the patient

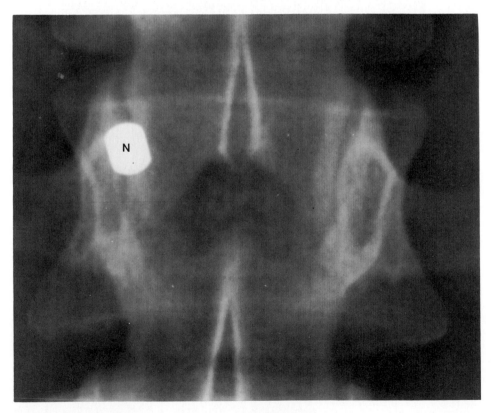

FIG. 3.9 Fluoroscopic spot film shows the hub of a 3½-inch needle (N) which has been directed vertically down to the left L4–L5 facet joint with the patient prone on the fluoroscopic table.

prone or minimally oblique on the fluoroscopic table, and a 3½-inch, 22-gauge needle has been directed into the joint (Fig. 3.9), intra-articular needle placement is confirmed by injecting a small amount (0.5 ml) of water-soluble contrast material (Reno-M-60®) (Figs. 3.10–3.12). Following successful placement of the needle tip, the joint is blocked by injecting 15 mg depo-Medrol® suspension and 2–4 ml 1 percent lidocaine solution.

Approximately two-thirds of patients with symptomatic lumbar facet arthropathy will respond to injection of the affected joint with relief of their entire pain complex within 5 min of injection (Table 3.2). On occasion, joint distention during the initial injection will reproduce the symptoms, which then disappear within 5 min.

A significant number of patients with symptomatic lumbar facet arthropathy remain asymptomatic after 10 days—2 weeks following injection (Table 3.2). This is presumably due to atrophy and retraction of the synovial-adipose villi from the joint caused by local steroid effect. Anatomic studies have shown that these synovial structures can be damaged by abnormal facet joints, and presumably can be the cause of both local and referred pain in the facet syndrome.[6, 14] Those patients who report initial pain relief that lasts for several weeks, followed by recurrent pain, may be candidates for a single attempt at reinjection on the premise that an inadequate steroid dose may have been administered in the initial injection.

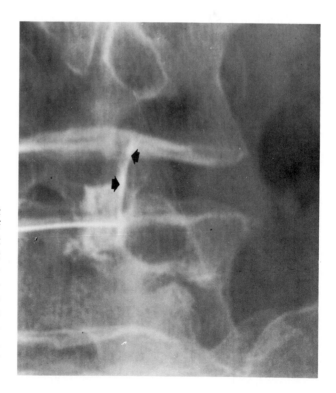

FIG. 3.10 Fluoroscopic spot film after injection of less than 0.5 ml contrast into the right L4–L5 facet joint. Contrast is seen between the articular cartilages (arrows). (With permission from Carrera, GF: Lumbar facet joint injection in low back pain and sciatica (I) and (II). Radiology 136:661–667, 1980.)

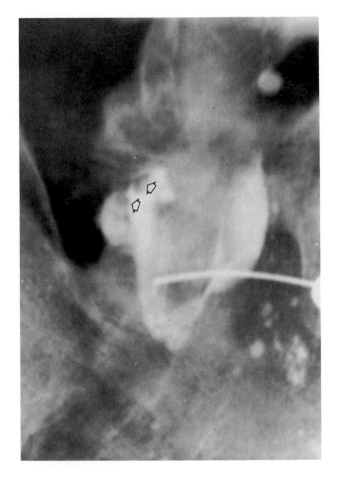

FIG. 3.11 Injection of 2.5 ml contrast outlines a capacious left L5–S1 facet joint. Irregular filling defects (arrows) in the superior margin of the joint represent the superior fat pad. Droplets of residual myelographic contrast overlie the spinal canal. (With permission from Carrera, GF: Lumbar facet joint injection in low back pain and sciatica (I) and (II). Radiology 136:661–667, 1980.)

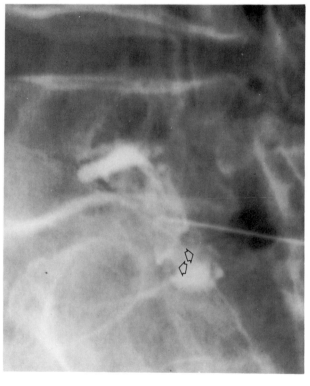

FIG. 3.12 Injection of 0.5 ml contrast material into a badly degenerated left L5–S1 facet joint shows extension of the joint capsule superiorly into the intervertebral foramen. Irregular filling defects caused by the inferior capsular fat pad (arrows) are seen. (With permission from Carrera, GF: Lumbar facet joint injection in low back pain and sciatica (I) and (II). Radiology 136:661–667, 1980.)

TABLE 3.2 Results of facet block in patients with clinically suspected facet syndrome

Number of patients	75
Immediate relief	51
Remain asymptomatic (6 months)	19
Reinjection (6 weeks—6 months)	10
Relief after reinjection	4

CONCLUSION

Pain referred from arthritic lumbar facet joints has remained a vexing diagnostic and therapeutic problem in patients with mechanical backache. Prior to CT, effective diagnosis of patients with abnormal lumbar facet joints was difficult and frequently frustrating. The clinical diagnosis of symptomatic lumbar facet arthropathy was similarly difficult and frequently inaccurate. High-resolution CT employing appropriate techniques for evaluating bony structures, performed as part of a standard examination of the spine and its contents in patients with backache and sciatica, effectively identifies a substantial population of patients with abnormal lumbar facet joints. A wide range of abnormalities ranging from mild hypertrophy and osteophyte formation to severe articular damage with erosions and profound reactive sclerosis can be easily evaluated on CT images.

Once this population of patients has been identified, it is the responsibility of the diagnostician to further test for symptomatic lumbar facet arthropathy using the more specific technique of intra-articular facet block. (Table 3.3) Although this technique has been employed for many years by clinicians, it is usually done without the benefit of fluoroscopic control by an experienced arthrographer. Accurate, intra-articular placement of the needle tip ensures that the relief (or lack of relief) of the patient's symptoms is an accurate test for symptomatic facet arthropathy.

TABLE 3.3 Correlation between CT and facet block in 53 patients

		Facet Block	
		Positive	**Negative**
	Positive	33	12
CT Scan			
	Negative	1	7

The presence of richly innervated synovial-adipose villi between articulating cartilages in normal individuals, and the demonstration of abnormalities of these structures due to mechanical trauma from abnormal joints, provides an anatomic rationale for treatment of symptomatic lumbar facet joints with local cortico-steroids. Intra-articular steroid suspension will cause atrophy and retraction of the adipose villi, thus removing the cause of pain from the joint. This phenomenon most likely accounts for the significant percentage of patients deriving long-term relief from a single injection of cortico-steroid suspension into an arthritic facet joint.

Even in patients who do not respond to facet injection with long-term relief, immediate relief of all symptoms after injection with local anesthetic solution provides a direct diagnostic examination for symptomatic lumbar facet arthropathy. The combination of CT examination and fluoroscopically controlled facet block, therefore, provides an effective and safe means for identifying patients with abnormal lumbar facet joints and testing those patients for symptomatic lumbar facet arthropathy.

References

1. Carrera GF, Williams AL, Haughton VM: Computed tomography in sciatica. Radiology 137:433, 1980.
2. Carrera GF, Haughton VM, Syvertsen A, Williams AL: Computed tomography of the lumbar facet joints. Radiology 134:145, 1980.
3. Badgley CE: Articular facets in relation to low back pain and sciatic-radiation. J Bone Joint Surg 23:481–496, 1941.
4. Ghormley RK: Low back pain with special reference to the articular facets, with presentation of an operative procedure. JAMA 101:1773–1777, 1933.
5. Inman VT and Saunders JBDM: The clinico-anatomical aspects of the lumbosacral region. Radiology 38:669–678, 1942.
6. Oppenheimer A: Diseases of the apophyseal (intervertebral) articulations. J Bone Joint Surg 20:285–313, 1938.
7. Mooney V, Robertson J: The facet syndrome. Clin Orthop Relat Res 115:149–156, 1976.
8. Williams AL, Haughton VM, Syvertsen A: Computed tomography in the diagnosis of herniated nucleus pulposus. Radiology 135:95, 1980.
9. Lee BCV, Kazam E, Newman AD: Computed tomography of the spine and spinal cord. Radiology 128:95, 1978.
10. Sheldon JJ, Sersland T, Leborgne J: Computed tomography of the lower lumbar vertebral column. Radiology 124:113, 1977.
11. Carrera GF: Lumbar facet joint injection in low back pain and sciatica (I) and (II). Radiology 136:661–667, 1980.
12. Carrera GF: Lumbar facet arthrography and injection in low back pain. Wis Med J (Symposium on Low Back Pain) 78 #12:35–37, 1979.
13. Lewin T, Moffett B, Viidik A: Morphology of the lumbar synovial intervertebral joints. Acta Morphol Neurol Scand 4:299–319, 1962.
14. Hadley LA: Anatomico-roentgenographic studies of the posterior spinal articulations. AJR 86:270–276, 1961.

15. Pedersen HE, Blunck CFJ, Gardener E: Anatomy of lumbosacral posterior rami and meningeal branches of spinal nerves (sinu-vertebral nerves) with experimental study of their function. J Bone Joint Surg 38A:377–391, 1956.

16. Stillwell DL Jr.: Nerve supply of vertebral column and its associated structures in the monkey. Anat Res 125:139–169, 1956.

17. Genant HK: Computed tomography of the lumbar spine: Technical considerations. pp. 23–52. In Genant HK, Chafety N, Helms CA, Eds.: Computed Tomography of the Lumbar Spine. Univ. of California Press, Berkeley, 1982.

4 Spinal Neoplasms

DAVID L. DANIELS

Since 1978, we have evaluated more than 50 patients with spinal tumors using computed tomography (CT) at Milwaukee County General and Froedtert Memorial Lutheran Hospitals. CT has proven to be complementary to myelography in characterizing tumors.

As compared to myelography, CT has many advantages. CT better defines a tumor's compartment (intramedullary, extramedullary, and intradural or extradural), a tumor's extension (epidural, osseous, and paraspinal), and other features of the tumor (calcification and hyperostosis of adjacent bone). With CT, tumors can be distinguished usually from nonneoplastic processes (syrinx, cyst) with similar myelographic appearances. CT also can be used to follow tumors and evaluate treatment. CT also can provide adequate images of a spinal tumor after a suboptimal metrizamide myelogram, in which for technical reasons, opacification of the subarachnoid space was inadequate.

TECHNIQUE

Symptoms suggesting intraspinal neoplasms such as back pain, a neurologic deficit or constitutional symptoms (weight loss, anorexia, etc.) cannot usually be localized precisely to one or two spinal levels. Therefore, in most patients with intraspinal neoplasms, myelography (metrizamide or gas) is needed initially for localization. If CT imaging follows within 3 hours of metrizamide myelography, the subarachnoid space is adequately enhanced for CT. If not, metrizamide is intrathecally injected in a "low dose" of 4 to 5 ml at 170 mg/ml to delineate an intramedullary or intradural-extramedullary tumor that narrows the subarachnoid space. Intravenous contrast agent (300 ml of 30 percent iodinated contrast agent) can be used to visualize enhancing intradural-extramedullary lesions such as meningioma, neurofibroma, or arteriovenous malformation and intramedullary lesions when intrathecal metrizamide is not present. In most cases, intravenous contrast agent is not necessary to evaluate extradural tumors.

53

Density measurements will not be stressed due to their variability when scans are obtained at different times after contrast administration and their inaccuracy when a small body calibration is used. However, density measurements can be used to distinguish cystic and solid masses in many cases.

Technical factors for CT scanning in spinal tumors include a lateral localizer scan and small-body calibration or target reconstruction. Five-millimeter-thick sections, zero degrees gantry angulation and reconstructed images are used to evaluate larger lesions; 1.5-mm-thick sections and a gantry angle perpendicular to the spine are used in smaller lesions.

INTRAMEDULLARY NEOPLASMS

Intramedullary neoplasms cause fusiform enlargement of cord contours and a decrease in the size of the adjacent subarachnoid space. Cord edema and glial cell infiltration lower the density of the enlarged cord and decrease the contrast between the cord and the subarachnoid space.[1] Due to these changes, the intramedullary neoplasm can be difficult to visualize with CT. Intrathecal enhancement with metrizamide usually is necessary for optimal demonstration of the expanded cord.

Ependymoma is the most frequent intramedullary neoplasm.[1-5] It occurs most commonly at the conus medullaris, where ependymal cells lining the central canal are numerous. The tumor can extend along the filum terminale or into the neural foramina. The contrast enhancement is minimal and observed near the central canal in some cases (Fig. 4.1). Pressure erosion by expanding tumor can cause spinal canal enlargement, posterior vertebral body scalloping, and lamina thinning (Fig. 4.2). Calcification is rare in ependymoma.

Glial tumors such as astrocytoma and glioblastoma are the next most frequent intramedullary neoplasms (Figs. 4.3, 4.4).[1-5] They show no predilection for a specific area. Contrast enhancement usually is minimal although a case of a markedly enhancing astrocytoma has been reported.[6] Calcification is rare. Cysts may be present but are difficult to identify due to adjacent low-density glial infiltration of the cord.

Hemangioblastoma is the next most common intramedullary neoplasm.[1] It is most often found in the cervical and thoracic regions. The tumor may show marked contrast enhancement (Fig. 4.5).[1, 4]

Other intramedullary masses include metastasis (especially lung carcinoma, melanoma, lymphoma) and lipoma. Intramedullary metastatic lesions usually produce enlargement of the cord without a characteristic morphologic appearance or enhancement pattern (Fig. 4.6). Metastatic medulloblastoma, a rare intramedullary lesion, does not have a characteristic CT appearance.[7] Lipoma with a CT number between −20 and −100 Hounsfield Units (HU) can be diagnosed by CT.[8]

Nonneoplastic processes that can enlarge the spinal cord are cyst (Figs. 4.7, 4.8), hematoma (Fig. 4.9), and cord edema from trauma, radiation, or multiple

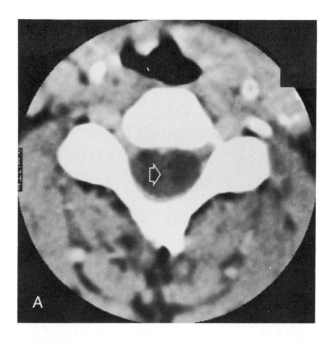

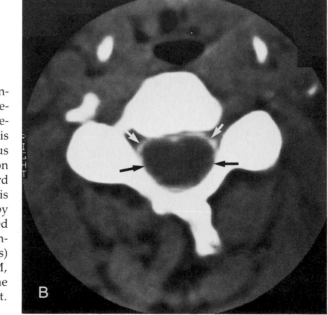

FIG. 4.1 Cervical ependymoma. Central ill-defined contrast enhancement (open arrow) is present after intravenous contrast administration (A). The enlarged cord contour not defined in A is outlined (black arrows) by the intrathecally enhanced and narrowed subarachnoid space (white arrows) in B. (From Haughton VM, Williams AL: CT of the Spine. CV Mosby Co., St. Louis, 1982.)

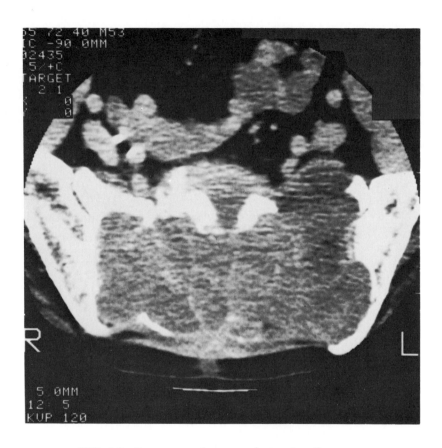

FIG. 4.2   Large ependymoma destroying the sacrum.

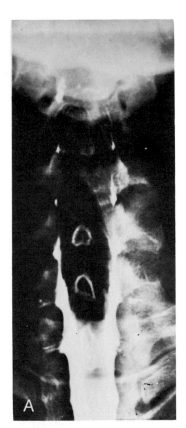

FIG. 4.3 Cervical astrocytoma. The cord is enlarged in the pantopaque myelogram (A) and in axial section (B). The density (43 HU) at the region of the tumor did not suggest cyst. Residual pantopaque (arrows) demarcates the tumor's contour in B.

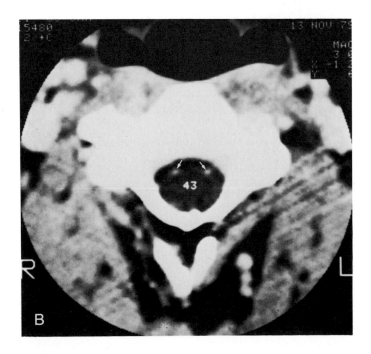

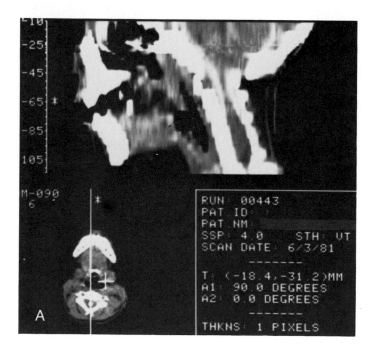

FIG. 4.4   Astrocytoma. The lower cervical intramedullary neoplasm is demonstrated in sagittal (A) and coronal (B) reconstructed images with intrathecal metrizamide.

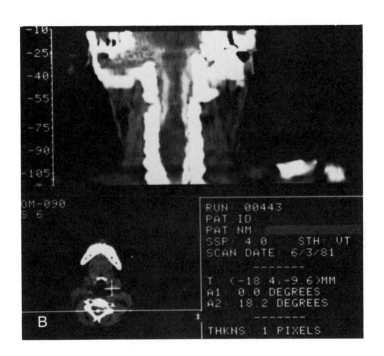

FIG. 4.4 (cont.)

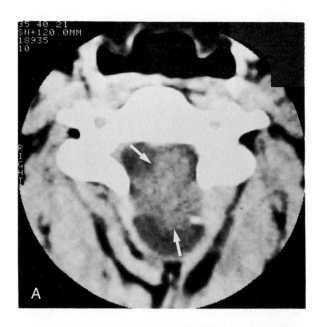

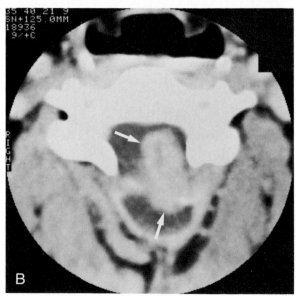

FIG. 4.5 Cord hemangioblastoma. The hemangioblastoma (arrows) markedly and homogeneously enhances without (A) and with (B) intravenous contrast medium. A pseudomeningocele is present at the site of a previous laminectomy. (From Haughton VM, Williams, AL: CT of the Spine. CV Mosby Co., St. Louis, 1982.)

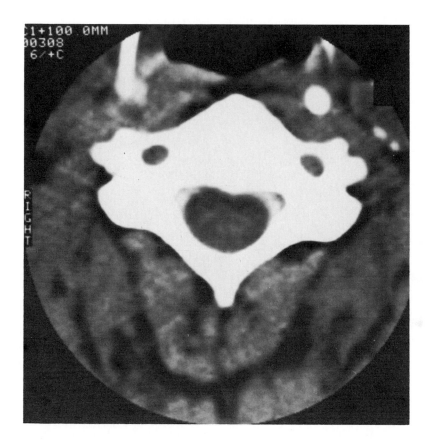

FIG. 4.6   Intramedullary metastatic lesion. A metastatic lung lesion has enlarged the lower cervical cord contour outlined by intrathecal metrizamide. (From Haughton VM, Williams, AL: CT of the Spine. CV Mosby Co., St. Louis, 1982.)

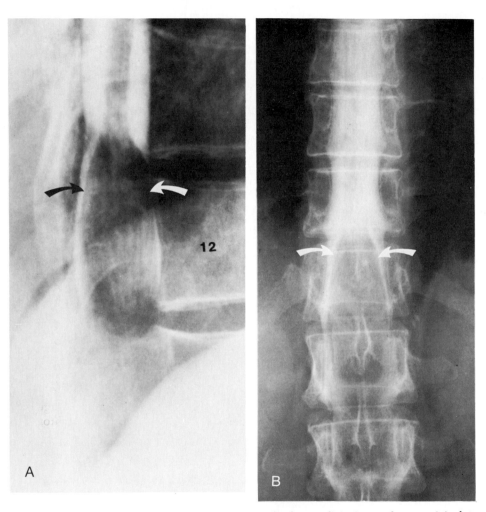

FIG. 4.7 Thoracic intramedullary cyst (syringohydromyelia). (curved arrows) in lateral (A) and AP (B) metrizamide myelogram films.

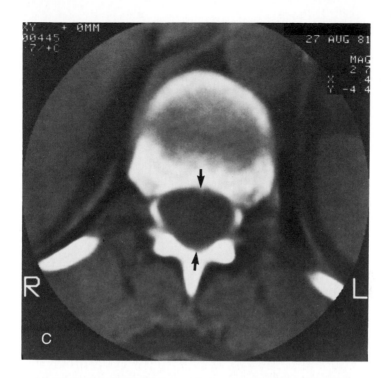

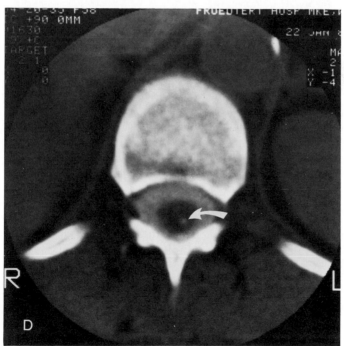

FIG. 4.7 (cont.)   The cyst with a density of 15 HU narrowed the subarachnoid space at T12 in metrizamide-enhanced CT (C). Six months after the cyst was shunted (curved arrow in D), the cord is normal sized.

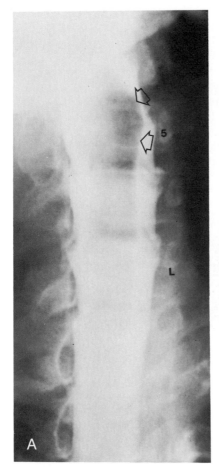

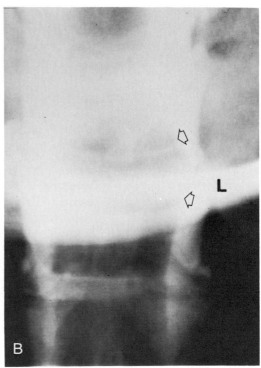

FIG. 4.8 Cervical intramedullary cyst. The midcervical cord is focally enlarged on the left (open arrows) in oblique and magnification myelogram films and an axial CT with intrathecal metrizamide.

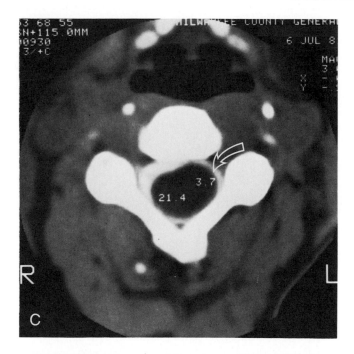

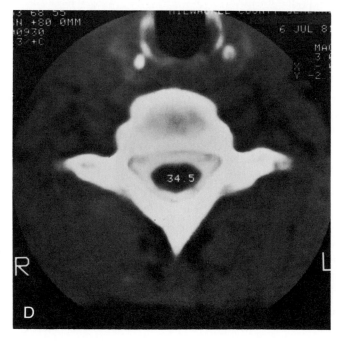

FIG. 4.8 (cont.)   The density of the focal area of enlargement (4 HU) in CT is less than the density of the normal cervical cord (35 HU) in D. At surgery the localized area of cord enlargement was a cyst.

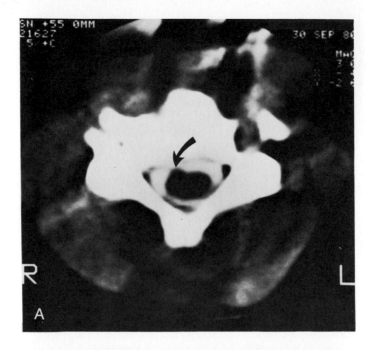

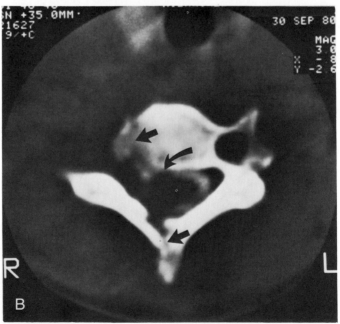

FIG. 4.9 Cervical cord hematoma and/or edema. Midcervical right sided localized cord enlargement (curved arrows) in axial images (A,B) with intrathecal metrizamide. Vertebral body and lamina fractures (straight arrows) status post gunshot wound is noted on the right in B.

sclerosis. These processes may be difficult to distinguish reliably from neoplasms. A large intramedullary cyst can have nearly the same density as a tumor. However, a mass with a density of 0 to 20 HU suggests cyst or cystic tumor (normal cord density is 30 to 40 HU). A central, well-defined, low-density area in an enlarged cord suggests syringohydromyelia. The diagnosis of syringohydromyelia is confirmed by a change in cord size in a gas myelogram performed in two positions.[9]

INTRADURAL EXTRAMEDULLARY NEOPLASMS

Neurofibromas, meningiomas, and lipomas are the most common intradural-extramedullary tumors.[1] Neurofibromas are solid tumors that arise from the epineurium of nerve roots and nerves. They occur throughout the spine with the same frequency in men and women.[5] Bone changes are common and include enlargement of the vertebral canal and/or neural foramina, erosion of pedicles, thinning of lamina, and scalloping of the posterior margin of vertebral bodies (Fig. 4.10). A large neurofibroma can involve more than one vertebral level. A neurofibroma is slightly more dense than the spinal cord and usually shows moderate homogeneous enhancement after intravenous contrast administration (Fig. 4.11). Calcification in a neurofibroma is rare. If the tumor is large and obliterates the subarachnoid space, intrathecal metrizamide will be needed to demarcate the tumor and displaced cord. CT effectively identifies intradural neurofibromas after intrathecal or intravenous contrast administration (Fig. 4.12) and the intradural and extradural components of a "dumbbell" neurofibroma (Fig. 4.13).[4] An anomalous dural sac and root sheath can mimic the appearance of a mass such as a neurofibroma in CT (Fig. 4.14).

Slightly less frequent than neurofibromas are spinal meningiomas that occur most commonly in the thoracic spine in females older than 40 years.[5] Meningiomas are solid, more dense than the spinal cord, and often contain calcification that can vary from punctate to globular (Fig. 4.15).[1, 4] Hyperostosis is a characteristic but uncommon feature of a meningioma (Fig. 4.16). Moderate contrast enhancement after intravenous contrast administration is typical of meningioma (Fig. 4.15) unless the mass is densely calcified. Extradural extension occurs uncommonly (Fig. 4.17). If the mass obliterates the subarachnoid space, intrathecal enhancement may be needed to demonstrate the mass.

Lipomas are more common in the filum terminale than in the cord or epidural space.[1] They can extend over a number of spine segments and be associated with an enlarged spinal canal, meningocele, and tethered cord.[1, 5] A lipoma has a characteristic CT appearance. It is sharply defined, less dense (-20 to -100 HU) than CSF,[4, 8] and not enhancing (Figs. 4.18, 4.19). It can be identified without intrathecal enhancement. Intrathecal contrast agent, however, may be necessary to evaluate an associated meningocele.[1]

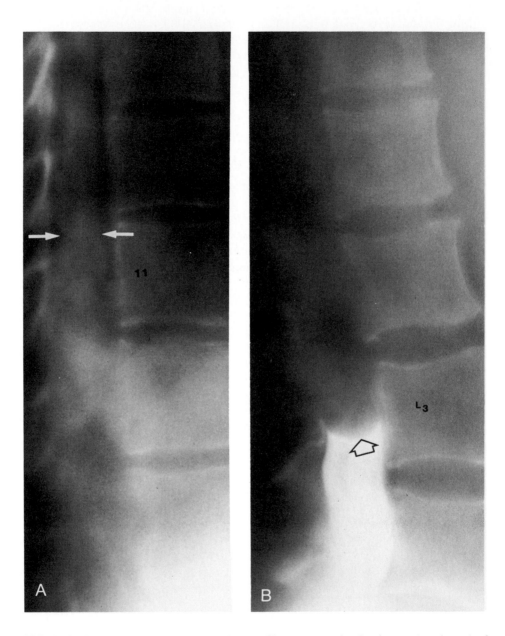

FIG. 4.10   Large intra- and extradural neurofibroma completely obstructing the spinal canal. The mass is defined superiorly (arrows) with gas at T11 and inferiorly (open arrow) with metrizamide at L3 on lateral polytomographic films (A,B).

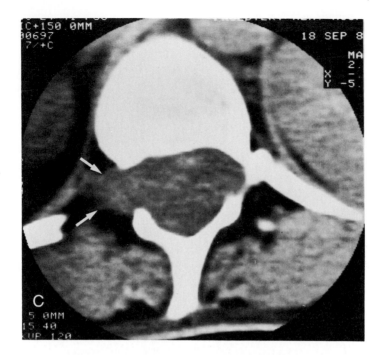

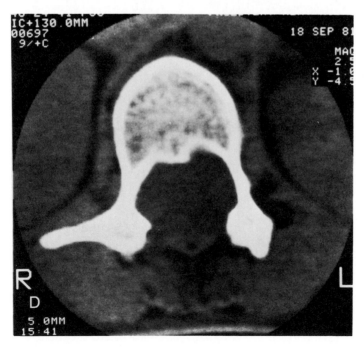

FIG. 4.10 (cont.) Intra- and extraspinal (arrows) tumor is present at T12 in axial CT section (C). Spinal deformity consists of an enlarged spinal canal, thin pedicles and a scalloped posterior vertebral body in D.

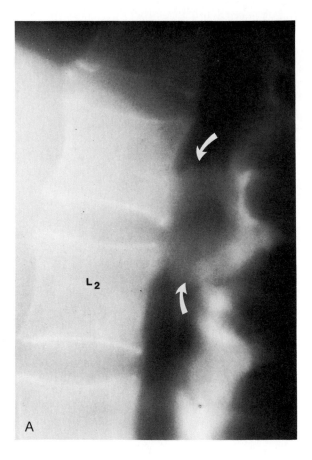

FIG. 4.11 Neurofibroma. A lumbar soft-tissue mass's superior and inferior borders (curved arrows) are defined by gas in a lateral polytomographic film (A).

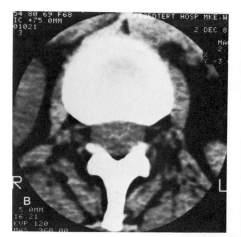
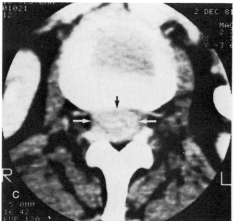
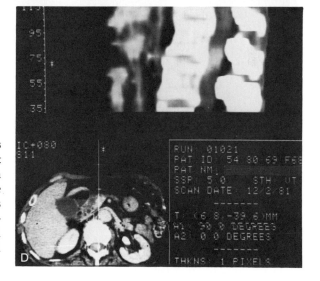

FIG. 4.11 (cont.) The mass's homogeneous enhancement (arrows) distinguishes it from other dural sac contents in the corresponding CT images without (B) and with (C) intravenous contrast agent and in a sagittal reconstructed image (D).

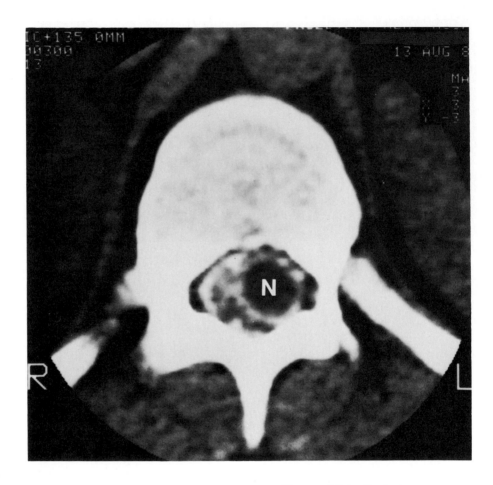

FIG. 4.12 Intradural neurofibroma. The neurofibroma (N) is displacing nerve roots to the right in an intrathecally enhanced axial CT scan at T12.

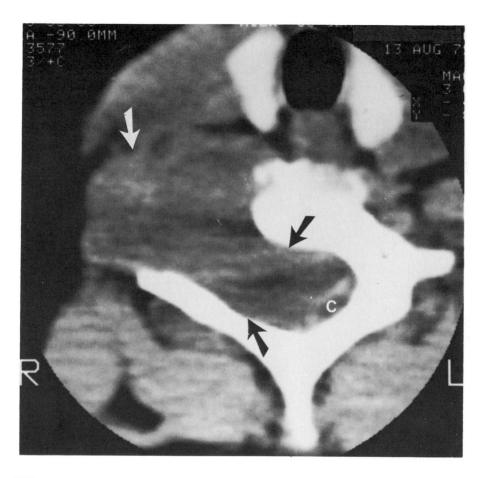

FIG. 4.13 "Dumbbell"-shaped neurofibroma. A large neurofibroma at the cervical-thoracic junction completely obstructed the spinal canal in a metrizamide myelogram. CT after the myelogram demonstrates large intra- and extradural components of the mass (arrows), an enlarged right C7 neural foramen, and the cervical cord (C) displaced and incompletely defined by intrathecal metrizamide. (From Haughton VM, Williams AL: CT of the Spine. CV Mosby Co., St. Louis, 1982.)

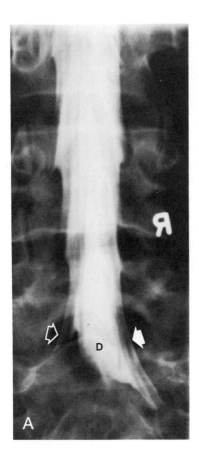

FIG. 4.14 Anomalous dural sac and root sheath. The anomalous dural sac (D) suggests a soft-tissue mass in axial CT (A) but is identified as dural sac (D) in a metrizamide myelogram (B). The S1 root sheath (open arrows) is visualized in both studies. Right-sided conjoined roots (closed arrow) are present in the myelogram.

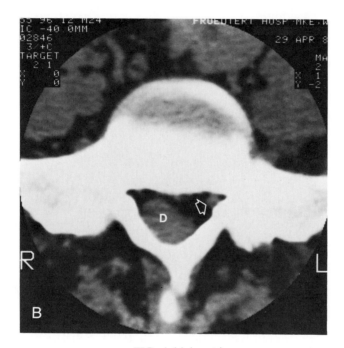

FIG. 4.14 (cont.)

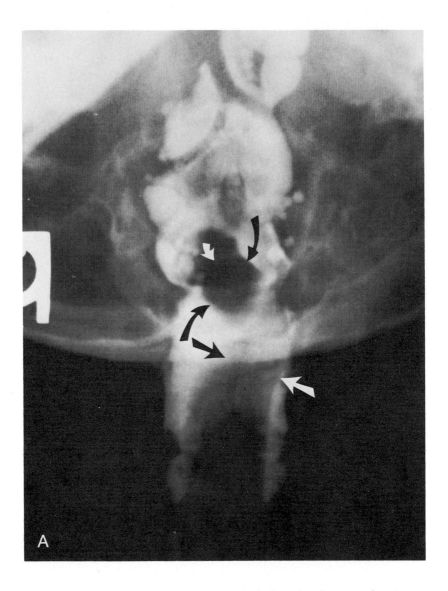

FIG. 4.15 Cervical meningioma that has calcified and enhances after intravenous contrast mediu. The intradural and extramedullary mass (curved arrows) displaces the upper cervical cord (straight arrows) in a frontal film from a pantopaque myelogram (A).

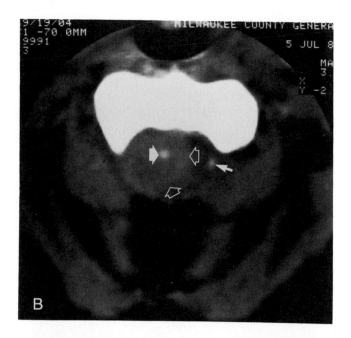

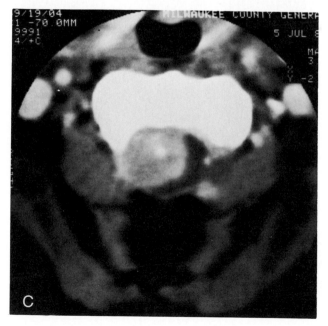

FIG. 4.15 (cont.) The mass (open arrows) is focally calcified (wide closed arrow) in axial CT (B) at C2 and homogeneously enhances after intravenous contrast administration in CT (C). Some residual pantopaque (thin closed arrow) is present in B. ((B) and (C) from Haughton VM, Williams AL: CT of the Spine, CV Mosby Co., St. Louis, 1982.)

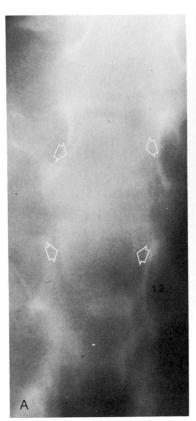
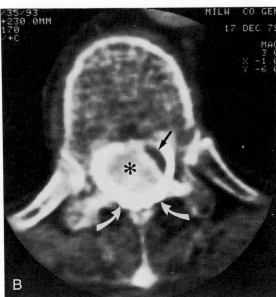

FIG. 4.16 Meningioma. The dense tumor (open arrows) completely obstructs the thoracic canal at T11–T12 in an anteroposterior polytomographic film from a gas myelogram (A). In axial CT (B), the meningioma (*) does not enhance after intravenous contrast administration, and is associated with hyperostosis (curved arrows) of the spinal canal. The thoracic cord (straight arrow) is displaced and compressed in B. ((B) from Haughton VM, Williams AL: CT of the Spine. CV Mosby Co., St. Louis, 1982.)

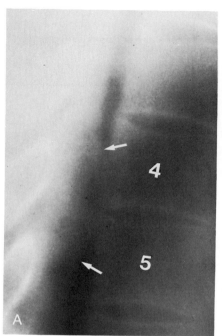

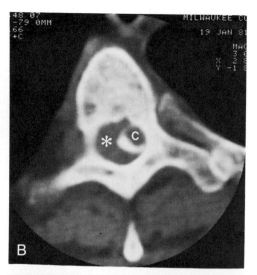

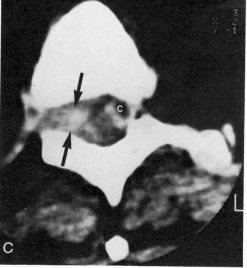

FIG. 4.17 Thoracic meningioma. In gas myelography (A) the cord appeared wide (arrows) at T4–T5. CT (B, C) shows that the cord (C) and dural sac are displaced by extradural tumor (*) that has some psammomatous calcification (arrows) (C). At surgery a meningioma having small intradural and large extradural components was found. ((B) from Haughton VM, Williams AL: CT of the Spine. CV Mosby Co., St. Louis, 1982.)

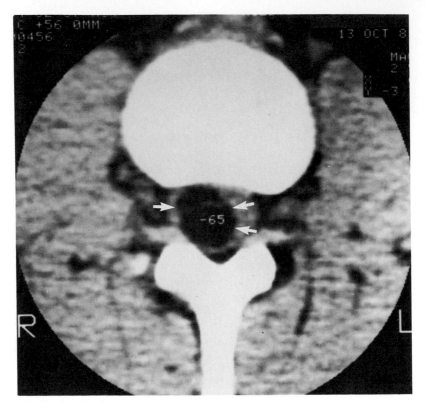

FIG. 4.18 Intradural lipoma. An upper lumbar lipoma of fat density (−65 HU) is sharply defined (arrows).

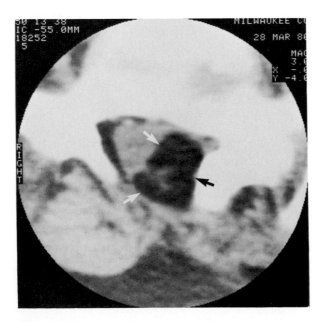

FIG. 4.19 Lipoma of filum terminale is sharply defined (arrows) at L5–S1. A large dysraphic defect at the neural arch is present. (From Haughton VM and Williams AL: CT of the Spine. CV Mosby Co., St. Louis, 1982.)

Dermoids and epidermoids usually occur at the conus or cauda equina (Fig. 4.20).[1, 5] These tumors do not have a characteristic CT appearance. Their diagnosis can be suggested if spina bifida, a pilonidal sinus, hypertrichosis, subcutaneous lipoma, or a midline draining sinus is present.

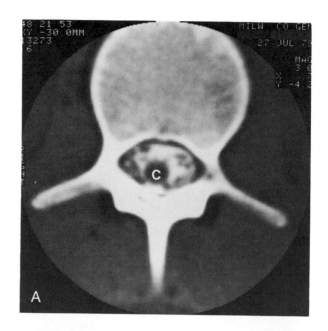

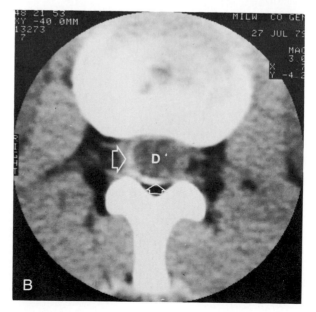

FIG. 4.20 Intradural dermoid. The lesion completely obstructed the spinal canal at L2 in a metrizamide myelogram. CT images (A,B) demonstrate a normal conus (C) at L1 and a dermoid (D) at L1–L2 incompletely outlined by metrizamide (open arrows). (From Haughton VM, Williams AL: CT of the Spine. CV Mosby Co., St. Louis, 1982.)

The differential diagnosis of intradural and extramedullary masses includes, among other things, neurenteric and arachnoid cysts (Figs. 4.21, 4.22). Cysts or cystic tumors can be distinguished from solid tumors. An extramedullary cyst has a density of 0 to 20 HU. If CT is performed after metrizamide enhancement of the subarachnoid space, a cyst that communicates with the subarachnoid space will become denser.

EXTRADURAL VERTEBRAL TUMORS

Extradural masses include benign and malignant tumors. The less common neoplasms are benign and include neurofibroma (Fig. 4.23), lipoma, dermoid, and epidermoid. These neoplasms usually have an intradural component and therefore are discussed above.[5] Neural foramen enlargement, typical of neurofibroma (Fig. 4.24), can also occur with other neoplasms, aneurysm (Fig.

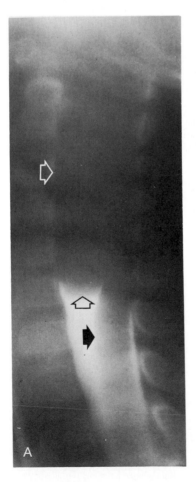

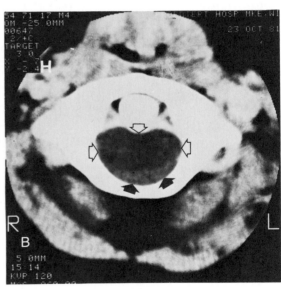

FIG. 4.21 Neurenteric cyst. A high-grade obstructing intradural and extramedullary upper cervical mass (open arrows) displaces the cervical cord (closed arrows) posteriorly, and widens the spinal canal in a lateral polytomographic film with intrathecal metrizamide (A) and in axial CT (B) at C1. The mass had a density of 10 HU consistent with cyst. At surgery a neurenteric cyst was found.

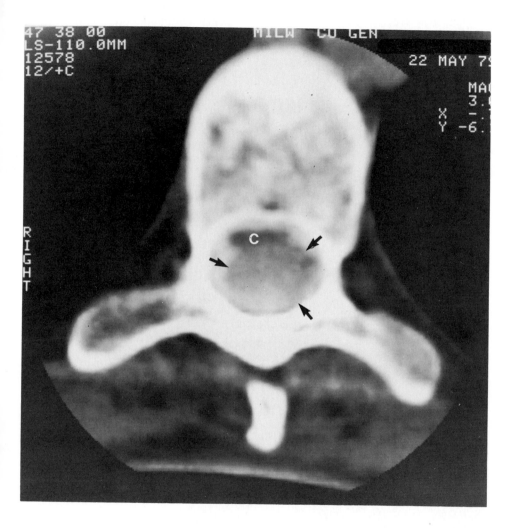

FIG. 4.22   Arachnoid cyst. Gas myelography suggested a posterior intradural mass at T9. A large intradural mass (arrows) partially enhanced with the intrathecal metrizamide displaces and compresses the thoracic cord (C) in axial CT at T9 with intrathecal metrizamide. (From Haughton VM, Williams AL: CT of the Spine. CV Mosby Co., St. Louis, 1982.)

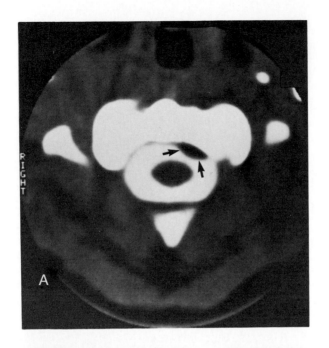

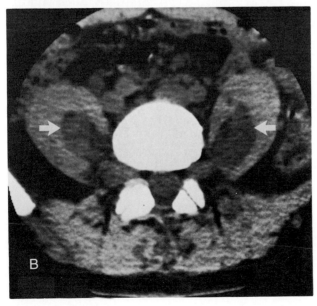

FIG. 4.23 Extradural neurofibromas in two patients. A small epidural neurofibroma (arrows) is sharply defined with intrathecal metrizamide at C2 in A. In B, large neurofibromas (arrows) are present in the lumbar neural foramina and psoas muscles.

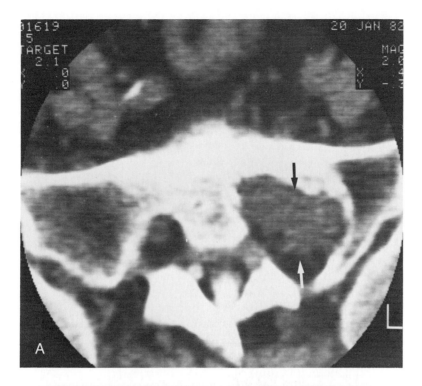

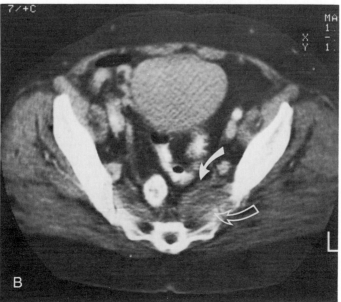

FIG. 4.24.   Sacral neurofibroma (arrows) expanding the left S2 neural foramen in A. A presacral component (curved arrows) is identified in B.

4.25), and meningocele (Fig. 4.26). To distinguish these processes, CT studies must be correlated with myelograms and angiograms.

Malignant epidural neoplasms typically obliterate epidural fat and destroy adjacent bone.[1] The soft-tissue mass in the spinal canal is defined by CT, especially if some epidural fat remains (Fig. 4.27).

Malignant osseous involvement with or without epidural tumor can be lytic, sclerotic (Figs. 4.28, 4.29), or a combination of lytic and sclerotic (Fig. 4.30). The margin of lytic bone destruction can be irregular and poorly defined (Fig. 4.27) to sharply defined (Figs. 4.31, 4.32). The margin can be sclerotic, especially in lymphoma (Fig. 4.33), osteosarcoma,[1, 11] or if the lesion has been treated with radiation or chemotherapy (Fig. 4.34). It is difficult to characterize the margin of a tumor that arises in abnormal bone such as pagetoid bone (Fig. 4.35).

CT offers an advantage over myelography in the study of epidural malignancies by demonstrating the extraosseous mass and better defining bone destruction (Fig. 4.36)[1, 4, 10] If surgical spinal cord decompression is a consideration in a high-grade obstructing lesion, the relationship of cord and tumor is better defined with CT than myelography (Fig. 4.37). In a spinal canal obstruction, a pathologic fracture fragment requiring surgical decompression can be distinguished by CT from epidural tumor that might be treated with radiation therapy (Fig. 4.38).

Processes that can simulate epidural tumors include herniated disc (Fig. 4.39), infection, hematoma, postoperative changes (Fig. 4.40), and cyst (Fig. 4.41). Discitis causing disc narrowing and vertebral end-plate destruction may be distinguished from tumor. The other processes seldom are associated with bone destruction. Some acute epidural hematomas can be identified accurately because their density is greater than 100 HU.[12]

Benign vertebral lesions such as osteochondroma, osteoblastoma, hemangioma, osteoid osteoma, and giant-cell tumor are less common than malignant ones.

Osteochondroma in the spine is uncommon. It may appear as a lesion of increased bone density exophytic to the spine.[1]

Osteoblastoma most frequently involves the posterior elements (Fig. 4.42). It appears in CT as an expansile lesion that destroys bone and encroaches on the spinal canal or neural foramina.[1, 13]

Hemangioma is a benign lesion most common in the vertebral body or the posterior elements of the lower thoracic or upper lumbar spine. Thick, longitudinal trabeculae are seen on the localizer image or a cross section in axial CT scans.[1] The lesion is sharply demarcated from normal bone (Fig. 4.43).

An osteoid osteoma in the spine appears as an area of sclerosis. The hypodense nidus may not be visualized due to partial volume averaging (Fig. 4.44).[1]

A giant-cell tumor is rare in the spine. CT typically demonstrates an expanding lytic lesion that initially involves the vertebral body. Aneurysmal bone cyst and osteoblastoma are other expanding lytic lesions, but they usually arise in the posterior elements.[14]

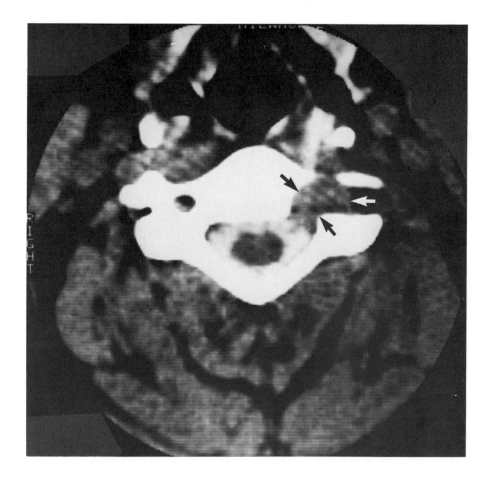

FIG. 4.25   Vertebral artery aneurysm. A soft-tissue mass (arrows) enlarging the left C4–C5 neural foramen in axial CT with intrathecal metrizamide.

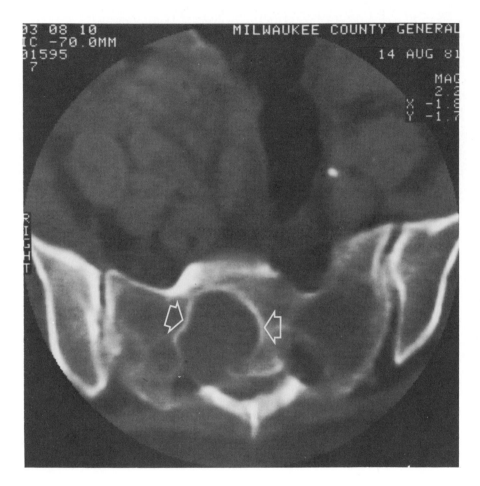

FIG. 4.26 Sacral meningocele. The right sacral foramen (arrows) is expanded. Metrizamide myelography demonstrated a meningocele.

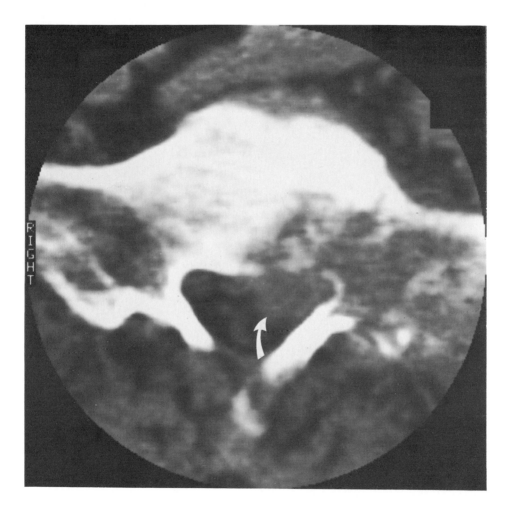

FIG. 4.27 Metastatic melanoma. The destructive left sacral tumor has an epidural component (curved arrow) that displaces epidural fat. The tumor's osseous margins are ill defined. (From Haughton VM, Williams AL: CT of the Spine. CV Mosby Co., St. Louis, 1982.)

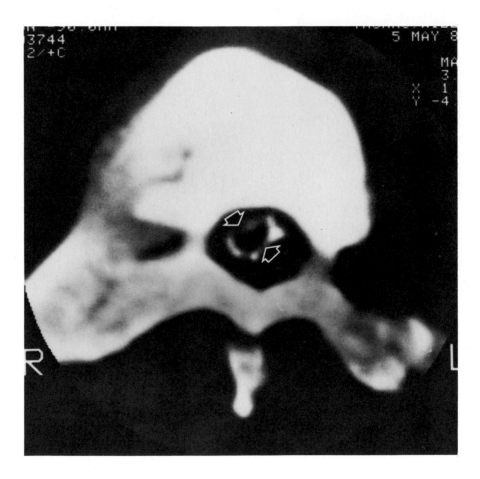

FIG. 4.28 Blastic prostatic metastasis involving the entire thoracic vertebra. Epidural tumor surrounds and indents (arrows) the dural sac with intrathecal metrizamide.

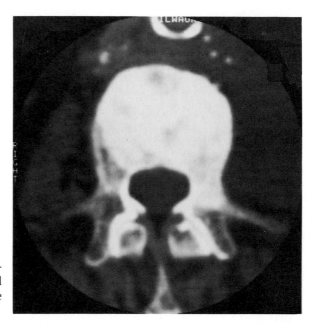

FIG. 4.29 Metastatic lymphoma. The L3 vertebral body and left pedicle are sclerotic.

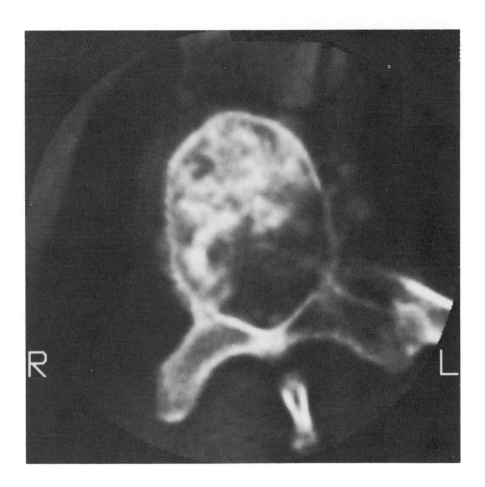

FIG. 4.30 Mixed lytic and sclerotic prostatic metastatic lesion.

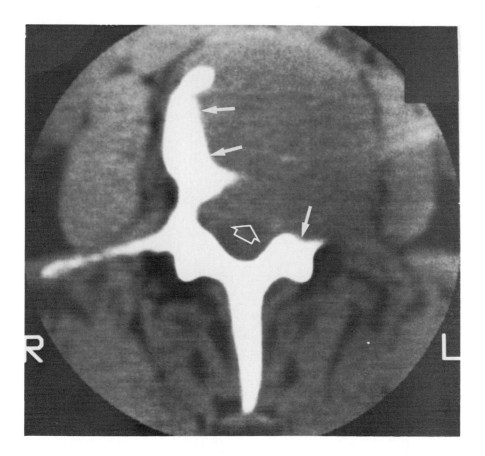

FIG. 4.31 Plasmacytoma. The tumor's lytic margins are sharply defined (closed arrows) at the L2 vertebral body and left pedicle. Epidural tumor (open arrow) is present.

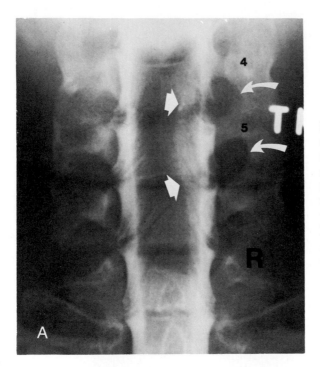

A

FIG. 4.32 Cervical chordoma (arrows) has enlarged the right C4–C5 and C5–C6 neural foramina (curved arrows) (film from a metrizamide myelogram (A)). The tumor (short arrows) has enlarged the right C4–C5 neural foramen (long arrows) and displaced the cord (C) and subarachnoid space to the left in axial CT (B). Marked bone destruction at either the clivus or sacral-coccygeal region would be more typical of chordoma.

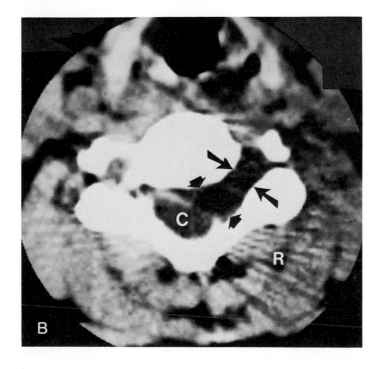

B

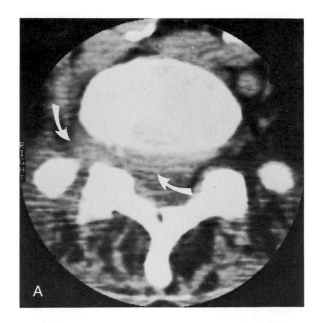

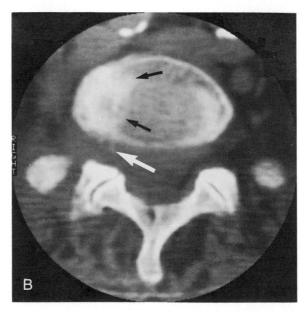

FIG. 4.33 Epidural lymphoma. The tumor obliterates epidural fat (arrows) at the right L5–S1 neural foramen in A. Cortical irregularity (white arrow) and sclerosis (black arrows) are present at the L5 vertebral body when the window is widened and bone detail examined in B. (From Haughton VM, Williams AL: CT of the Spine. CV Mosby Co., St. Louis, 1982.)

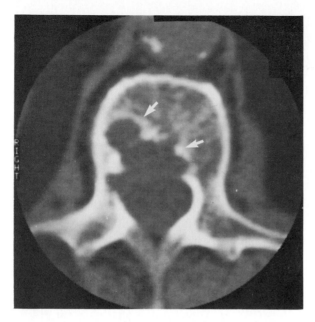

FIG. 4.34 Osteolytic lesion with a sclerotic border. This metastatic breast lesion after radiation therapy has sclerotic margins (arrows). (From Haughton VM, Williams AL: CT of the Spine. CV Mosby Co., St. Louis, 1982.)

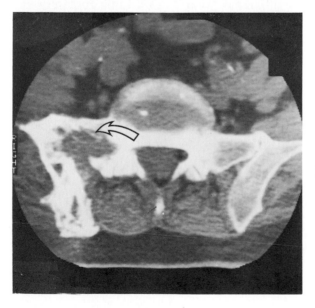

FIG. 4.35 Sarcoma (arrow) arising in pagetoid bone at the right hemipelvis. Serial CT scans showed progressive lysis of sclerotic bone from the sacral mass. (From Haughton VM, Williams AL: CT of the Spine. CV Mosby Co., St. Louis, 1982.)

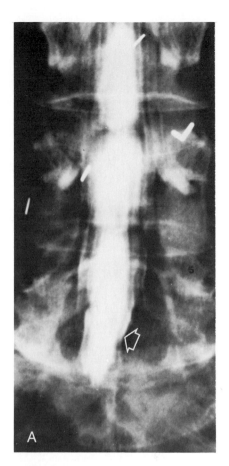

FIG. 4.36 Extradural lymphoma. The tumor minimally distorts the lower dural sac on the left (open arrow) in a metrizamide myelogram (A). Left-sided sacral destruction (curved arrow) and a presacral mass (closed arrow) are visualized in CT (B).

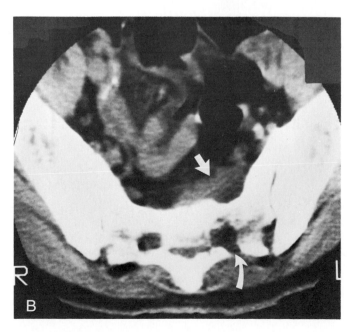

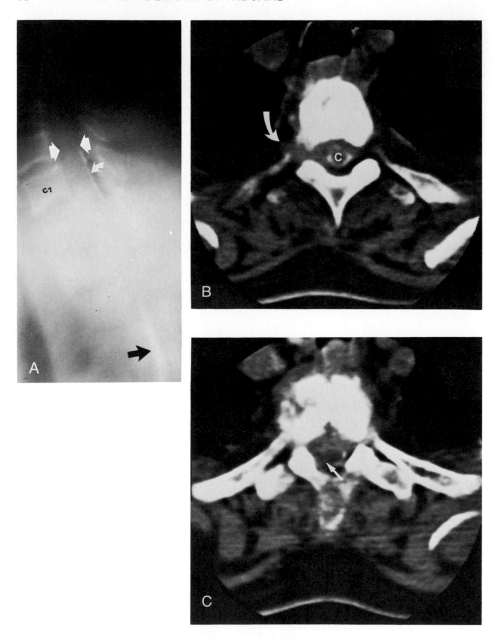

FIG. 4.37 High-grade obstructing epidural metastatic lesion. The tumor margins are defined superiorly by gas at C7–T1 and inferiorly by metrizamide (black arrow) at T3 in a lateral polytomographic film (A). The cervical cord (white arrows) is normal. A small amount of metrizamide (curved arrow) has gone above the obstructing lesion. In axial CT after the myelogram, tumor is identified at the right T3–T4 neural foramen (curved arrow (B)) and at the right ventral aspect of the spinal canal (straight arrow (C)) at T3. The thoracic cord (C) is not displaced at T3–T4.

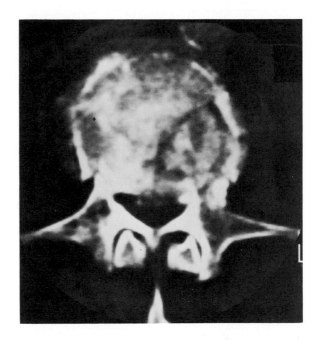

FIG. 4.38 Bone fragment obstructing the spinal canal at L3. The patient had a pathologic fracture from metastatic breast carcinoma.

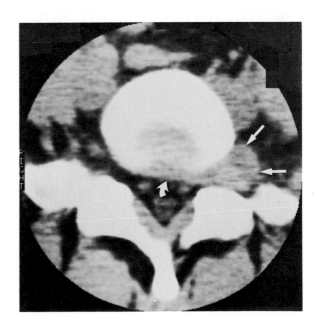

FIG. 4.39 Lateral L5–S1 herniated disc mimicking an extradural tumor. A soft-tissue mass (straight arrows) lateral to the left L5–S1 neural foramen is contiguous with the posterior disc margin (curved arrow). At surgery, the soft-tissue mass consisted of three free fragments. (From Haughton VM, Williams AL: CT of the Spine. CV Mosby Co., St. Louis, 1982.)

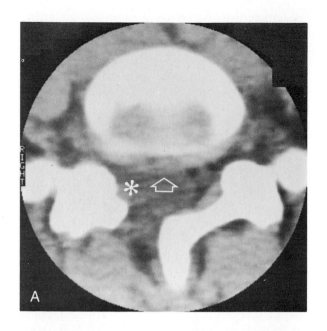

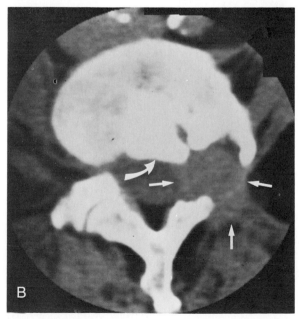

FIG. 4.40 Postoperative fibrosis in two patients. The epidural fat (*) is obliterated at the site of the previous laminectomy and disc mildly bulges posteriorly (open arrows) in A. In another patient (B), the patient has had an anterior interbody fusion (curved arrow) and a partial left facetectomy at L4–L5. Fibrous tissue (straight arrows) mimics the appearance of epidural tumor. ((A) From Haughton VM, Williams AL: CT of the Spine. CV Mosby Co., St. Louis, 1982.)

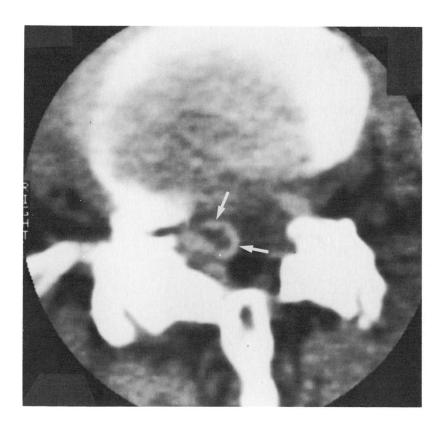

FIG. 4.41 Synovial cyst. The cyst is adjacent to the degenerated L4–L5 facet joint and has a calcified rim (arrows). A synovial cyst is associated with degenerative changes in a facet joint, nearly always at L3–L4. (From Haughton, VM, Williams AL: CT of the Spine. CV Mosby Co., St. Louis, 1982.)

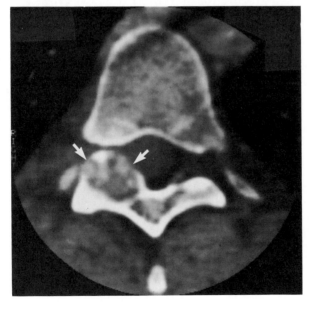

FIG. 4.42 Osteoblastoma (arrows) narrowing the right T8 neural foramen and the right side of the spinal canal. (From Haughton, VM, Williams AL: CT of the Spine, CV Mosby Co., St. Louis, 1982; case courtesy O. Petter Eldevik, M.D., Oslo.

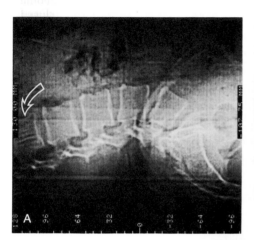

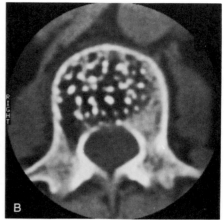

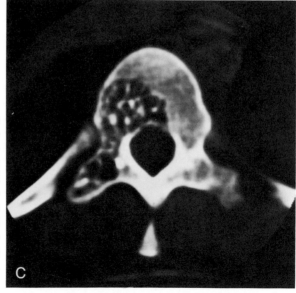

FIG. 4.43 Hemangiomas in two patients. The hemangiomas are visualized at L1 (curved arrow) in a localizer scan (A) and in axial section (B) in one patient and in an axial section (C) in another patient. Vertically coarse trabeculae and a sharp demarcation between normal and abnormal bone characterizes hemangioma. ((A),(B) from Haughton VM, Williams, AL: CT of the Spine. CV Mosby Co., St. Louis, 1982.

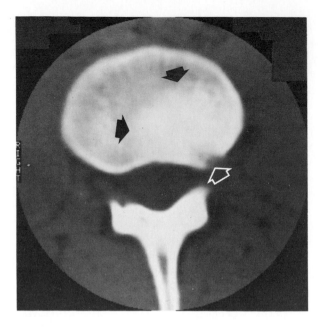

FIG. 4.44 Osteoid osteoma at L2. Focal sclerosis (closed arrows) and a hypodense nidus (open arrow) characterize osteoma. The nidus may not be visualized due to partial volume averaging. (From Haughton VM, Williams AL: CT of the Spine. CV Mosby Co., St. Louis, 1982.)

References

1. Haughton VM, Williams AL: CT of the Spine. CV Mosby Co., St. Louis, 1982.

2. Aubin ML, et al.: Computed tomography in 32 cases of intraspinal tumors. Neuroradiol 6:81–92, 1979.

3. Baleriaux-Waha D, et al.: CT of the adult spine with metrizamide. In Post MJD, Ed.: Radiologic Evaluation of the Spine: Current Advances with Emphasis on Computed Tomography. Masson, New York, 1880.

4. Nakagawa H, et al.: Computed tomography of intraspinal and paraspinal neoplasma. J Comput Assist Tomogr 1:377–390, 1977.

5. Taveras JM, Wood EH: Diagnostic Neuroradiology. Williams & Wilkins Co., Baltimore, 1976.

6. Handel S, Grossman R, Sukwar M: Computed tomography in the diagnosis of spinal cord astrocytoma. J Comput Assist Tomogr 2:226–228, 1978.

7. Fumpano BJ: Spinal intramedullary metastatic medulloblastoma. J Neurosurg 48:632–635, 1978.

8. Kaplans JO, Quenar RM: The occult tethered conus syndrome in the adult. Radiology 137:387–391, 1980.

9. Williams AL, Haughton VM: Gas myelography: Its current role in evaluation of the spine. In Post MJD, Ed.: Radiologic Evaluation of the Spine: Current Advances with Emphasis on Computed Tomography. Masson, New York, 1980.

10. Resjo IM, et al.: CT metrizamide myelography for intraspinal and paraspinal neoplasms in infants and children. AJR 132:367–372, 1979.

11. Harwood-Nash DC, Fitz CR: Computed tomography and the pediatric spine: Computed tomographic metrizamide myelography in children. In Post MJD, Ed.: Radiographic Evaluation of the Spine: Current Advances with Emphasis on Computed Tomography. Masson, New York, 1980.

12. Post MJD, et al.: CT diagnosis of spinal epidural hematoma. Am J Neuroradiol 3:190–192, 1982.

13. Nakagawa H, Mallis LI, Huang YP: Computed tomography of soft tissue masses related to the spinal column. In Post MJD, Ed.: Radiographic Evaluation of the Spine: Current Advances with Emphasis on Computed Tomography. Masson, New York, 1980.

14. Schwinger SR, et al.: Giant cell tumor of the cervico-thoracic spine. AJR 136:63–67, 1981.

5 Spine Trauma

PATRICK A. TURSKI

Traumatic injury to the spine and spinal cord is a serious medical problem with potential long-term social and economic consequences. The association of spine fractures and paraplegia was appreciated as early as 1600 BC by Egyptian physicians and recorded in the Edwin Smith Surgical Papyrus.[1] Recapitulating the rapid application of Roentgen's x-rays for the evaluation of spinal trauma, computed tomography was quickly utilized for examining patients with spine fractures.[2,3] The resulting axial CT image seemed ideal for evaluating the roughly circular osseous bony canal. Initial evaluations were limited by thick CT sections, long scan times, and difficulty in localizing and orienting the scan plane to the area of interest. Technologic advances have overcome these limitations and add new dimensions to computed tomography, further expanding its role in spine trauma. CT has already replaced pluridirectional tomography in many situations and is often the only radiologic procedure performed after the plain film exam.

TECHNIQUE

All CT investigations of the spine must begin with a system relating the scan plane to the area of interest. The most convenient method is a digital localizer image generated by the scanner x-ray source and detector system. This system allows display of the exact location of the CT slice in relation to the area of abnormality. If the scan plane is not optimal for demonstrating the pathologic process under investigation, it may be necessary to angle the gantry to obtain the desired plane.

The availability of thin CT sections (1.5–5.0 mm) has enabled detection of small minimally displaced fractures. Partial volume averaging is reduced with thin CT sections and only fractures that lie parallel to the scan plane are difficult to identify. A more conventional display of osseous anatomy may be obtained by employing multiplanar reformatting programs. The computer manipulation of axial CT data has been successfully applied to a variety of problems. A series of scans taken through a dislocated and fractured vertebra may be reformatted in sagittal and coronal planes, facilitating determination of the extent of fracture fragmentation and degree of dislocation. To obtain high-quality reformatted images a small table increment is desirable. For example, if 5.0-mm sections are obtained, a 2.0- or 3.0-mm table increment is preferred. When 1.5-mm collimation is utilized, a greater number of scans are required to cover the region of interest but spatial resolution improves and the reformatted images are more anatomic in appearance.[4]

The utilization of alternate algorithms (Target Review®) can reduce pixel size and increase bone detail considerably. Target images may also be used for multiplanar reformatting. The additional computer manipulation increases processing time and may not be practical in all situations.

The radiation dose for a CT examination varies with the type of scanner. In general, the radiation burden for spine CT is less than a comparable examination performed with pluridirectional tomography.[5, 6]

Intravenous contrast medium has not been generally utilized in CT examination of spine fractures. Its potential role in the assessment of injury to the spinal cord has not been explored. Certainly, associated soft-tissue injuries to the vascular system and genitourinary tract are better visualized on CT after the administration of intravenous contrast medium.

Intrathecal contrast material may be used to better define spinal canal soft-tissue contents (Fig. 5.1). Small amounts (3–5 cc 170 percent) of metrizamide, a water-soluble contrast medium, opacify the spinal canal adequately to outline the cord and to define its relationship to adjacent abnormalities.[7] Roub and Drayer[8] have also successfully employed oxygen to demonstrate a traumatic block.

Patients undergoing CT exams must be able to remain still during the scan sequence. Patient motion not only results in misregistration artifacts in the reformatted images but can result in a significant abnormality not being visualized due to motion artifact or movement of the abnormal region out of the plane of section. Therefore, the acutely traumatized patient may need sedation.

INDICATIONS

The initial radiologic investigation of a patient with suspected spine trauma remains the standard radiograph. Anteroposterior, lateral, oblique, coned-down views and specialized projections to visualize specific structures (e.g., the odontoid) should all be obtained when clinically indicated. Due to the high frequency of associated spine fractures remote from the primary injury site, the entire spine should be examined. For situations in which the patient is immediately transported to the scanner for intracranial examination, the digital localizer image may be used to screen the spine for major anatomic disruptions. When this technique is not satisfactory standard radiographs should be performed at the earliest possible opportunity.

Systematic comparisons of pluridirectional tomography and CT have been carried out to determine the optimal modality. Conclusions from these comparisons depend heavily on the capabilities of the scanner under consideration. CT sections of 13-mm thickness certainly do not compare as favorably

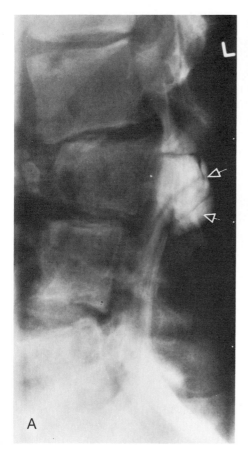

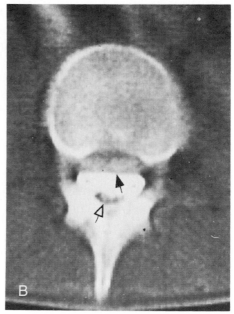

FIG. 5.1 Hyperflexion injury with comminuted fracture of L2. The lumbar metrizamide myelogram (A) reveals a pseudo-meningocele (open arrows) and compromise of the spinal canal from posteriorly displaced osseous fragments. Axial CT section (B) clearly defines the posteriorly displaced bony fragment (closed arrow) and intraspinal soft-tissue structures (open arrow).

as 1.5- or 5.0-mm CT sections. For example the spatial resolution of a 5.0-mm CT section is inferior to a pluridirectional tomogram. The CT section, however, provides superior contrast resolution and information regarding spinal canal compromise and soft-tissue injury. If a 1.5-mm section is obtained and processed by an alternate algorithm reducing pixel size (Target Imaging®), the spatial resolution can be greatly improved and approaches that obtained with pluridirectional tomography.

Pluridirectional tomography is easily performed in the anteroposterior plane. For lateral filming the patient must be turned into the decubitus position. If the spine is severely traumatized and unstable the turning of the patient into the decubitus position could have an adverse effect on the injured neural tissues.[9] The lateral filming permits visualization of fracture fragments in the sagittal plane but when compared to computed tomography is less accurate in evaluating spinal canal compromise.[6]

Another distinct advantage of computed tomography is that once the patient is positioned on the CT table there is usually no further manipulation of the patient. In the severely traumatized patient this is an important consideration. Even patients in traction can be scanned relatively simply. The traction apparatus can be passed through the scanner gantry and suspended over the edge of the scan table so that there is no disturbance of traction during the radiologic examination.

Fractures of the vertebral body are easily identified with either modality. However, computed tomography is more accurate in identifying comminuted fractures and defining the position of displaced fracture fragments. Fractures lying horizontally (i.e., parallel to the scan plane) may be missed by computed tomography due to partial volume averaging if thick CT sections are utilized. Similarly, fractures extending through the pedicles that are oriented in the transverse plane may be difficult to identify with CT. Fractures involving the lamina, spinous process, or lateral masses are more easily identified on computed tomography than on pluridirectional tomography and the orientation of the fracture fragments is clearer.[6, 9] In general, CT provides greater information than polytomography regarding the degree of fracture fragmentation and the orientation of fracture fragments.

The major advantage of computed tomography is rapid determination of the status of the spinal canal and its contents. Assessment of the posterior elements may be accomplished by either method but computed tomography is more effective. Pluridirectional tomography is still a valuable adjunct for the assessment of confusing osseous abnormalities, nondisplaced fractures, or fractures oriented in the axial plane.

CERVICAL SPINE

The occipito-atlanto-axial region is usually considered separately since it functions as an anatomic unit. Fractures and dislocations of this region have several unique characteristics. Axial CT sections provide the optimal view of the foramen magnum. Fractures of the occipital condyles and the margins of the foramen magnum are better identified by computed tomography than any other radiologic technique.[10]

Anterior occipito-atlanto dislocation is a severe injury that is rarely associated with survival and is sometimes difficult to diagnose radiographically. Powers et al.[11] determined that the ratio of the distance from the basion to the midpoint of the arch canal line (BC) to the distance from the opisthion to the posterior surface of the anterior arch of the atlas (OA) is normally less than 1. If the BC/OA ratio is greater than 1, the skull is dislocated anteriorly on the axis. The CT findings in atlanto-axial dislocation have not been reported but one would presume that contiguous sections would demonstrate an abrupt compromise of the spinal canal at the site of the dislocation with disruption of the articulating surfaces between the occipital condyles and superior portions of the lateral masses of C1. The BC/OA ratio may be applied to sagittal reformatted images.

Transversely oriented CT sections provide a better spatial understanding of burst type fractures of the atlas (Jefferson Fracture). The relationship of the fracture fragments to the cervical cord are readily appreciated. Fractures occur most often in the anterior arch (Fig. 5.2) and at the junction of the posterior arch and lateral masses. The usual injury is a blow to the top of the head with compression of the atlas from above by the occipital condyles and from below by the superior articulating surfaces of C2. The fracture fragments are typically displaced outward in a radial fashion.[12–14] Differentiation from congenital spondylolishthesis of the atlas is accomplished by recognizing that congenital lesions have smooth, well-corticated margins.[15]

The primary function of the atlanto-axial joint is rotation. Rotational subluxation and pathologic fixation of the atlanto-axial joint is an uncommon condition that usually presents clinically as torticollis after head trauma. Rinaldi et al.[17] emphasized that the relationship of the atlas to the axis is fixed in this condition and they move as a unit. The abnormal fixation may be demonstrated with computed tomography by having the patient turn his head to the right for one set of scans and to the left for a second set of scans.[16, 17] In a normal situation this maneuver results in the atlas rotating on the less-

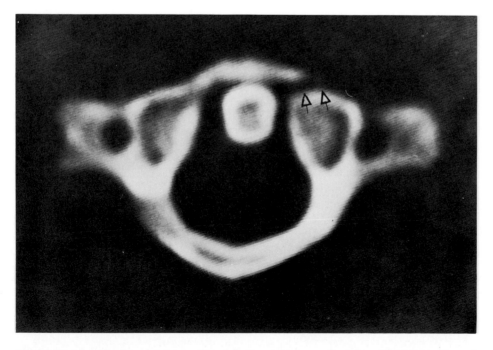

FIG. 5.2 Nondisplaced fracture through the anterior arch of the atlas (open arrows).

mobile axis. Although the pathophysiology remains elusive, Fielding and Hawkins[18] have proposed that reduction is hindered by swollen capsular and synovial tissue associated with muscle spasm. If reduction is not achieved in a relatively short time, fixation will occur secondary to capsular and ligamentous contracture.

Atlanto-axial dislocation occurs most often in conjunction with fracture of the odontoid. Hyperflexion and hyperextension are the most common causes of odontoid process fracture. The fracture is usually oriented transversely along the base of the dens or across the upper body. Axial CT sections are oriented parallel to the fracture plane and may demonstrate only a slight discontinuity of the cortex. Sagittal reformatted images are often necessary to clearly delineate the extent of injury. Fortunately, odontoid fractures are usually identified on the standard radiographs and the CT examination may be directed toward assessment of the cervical spinal canal and cord (Fig. 5.3).[9, 19]

Rarely traumatic dislocation may occur without dens fracture (Down's Syndrome, os odontoidium, rheumatoid arthritis). In these situations the odontoid may be abnormal or the transverse ligaments lax or disrupted. The dens should be within 3 mm of the posterior surface of the anterior arch of C1 in the adult and 5.0 mm in children.[20] Abnormal relationships between the anterior arch of the atlas and the odontoid can be demonstrated by axial CT sections.[14]

Fractures through the vertebral arch of the axis may be unilateral or bilateral. Compressive hyperextension with rotation is the probable mechanism of injury in the unilateral lesions. The much more common situation is bilateral arch fractures (hangman's fracture) usually the result of hyperextension of the skull on the upper cervical spine. The anatomic features include bilateral avulsion of the C2 vertebral arch through the pedicles with or without dislocation of C2 on C3. Since the fractures are usually oriented in vertical or oblique planes they are easily identified on axial CT sections (Fig. 5.4).[9, 10] Associated hematomas and soft-tissue swelling may also be identified.

Traumatic hyperflexion injuries to the lower cervical spine may be divided into fractures of the vertebral body, fractures of the vertebral arch, dislocations, and fracture dislocations.[20]

Vertebral Body

Simple margin fractures appear on CT as small discontinuities along the anterior superior or anterior inferior aspect of the body resulting from hyperextension or hyperflexion associated with compression. There is no compromise of the spinal canal. Axial compression results in a comminuted "burst" fracture. If the posterior fragments are displaced into the spinal canal, neurologic deficit may result. CT has an important function in this situation defining the multiple fracture lines and the degree of spinal canal compromise. Soft-tissue edema and hematoma may also be visualized on the CT images.[8] Fractures of the uncinate process and lateral hyperflexion compression fractures of the vertebral body have been described.[10]

Vertebral Arch

Fractures of the articular pillars are difficult to identify on plain films. Patients often complain of neck pain and on physical examination there is limitation of motion, tenderness, and muscle weakness. CT or pluridirectional tomography is usually necessary to identify these fractures. Axial CT sections demonstrate fractures oriented in the vertical plane. Compression fractures of the articular pillars may be difficult to identify on axial CT sections but oblique reformatted images may allow detection of these fractures. Fractures involving the lamina, spinous process, or transverse processes are clearly delineated on axial sections (Figs. 5.5 and 5.6). The degree of distraction of the fracture fragments is often better appreciated than on pluridirectional tomography.[9, 10, 22]

Dislocations and Fracture Dislocations

Hyperflexion injury may result in momentary dislocation with fracture, locked articular facets with fracture, or "teardrop" fracture dislocation. Hyperflexion sprain (momentary dislocation) is a temporary and partial dislocation of the apophyseal joints with rupture of the posterior ligaments and joint capsules. Approximately half of the patients will have associated fractures. Locked articular facets are the result of disruptive hyperflexion. Unilateral locked facet is often due to hyperflexion and rotation.[20] The CT diagnosis of locked facet may be difficult unless the sections are symmetric and the smallest collimation possible employed. In unilateral facet locking the joint surface of the inferior articular facet defines the posterior contour of the articular pillar and the posterior margin appears flat on axial CT sections. There is also vertebral body rotation.[9, 10, 22, 23] If the facet locking is bilateral, the spinal canal may be severely compromised and the posterior margins of both articular colums appear flattened on axial CT sections. "Teardrop" hyperflexion fracture-dislocation results in fracture of the anteroinferior aspect of the vertebral body. The apophyseal joints and the posterior portion of the vertebral disc are disrupted. The fracture fragment resembles a teardrop.[20] Computed tomography demonstrates comminuted "teardrop" fractures of the vertebral body better then conventional plain films. Spinal canal compromise and soft-tissue injury may also be seen. CT is less effective in demonstrating widened spinous processes or loss of vertebral body height secondary to "teardrop" fracture.

Coin et al.[23] described the CT findings in a series of patients who experienced diving type injuries to the cervical spine. They observed that vertical fractures involving the anterior margin of the spinal canal in association with fractures of the lamina (with or without displacement of fragments) were the most common. These injuries are presumed to be due to hyperflexion type stresses. A wedge fracture of the body was a frequently noted abnormality.

Hyperextension injuries may result in momentary dislocation, fracture-dislocation with fractured articular pillar or fracture-dislocation with comminution of the vertebral arch.[20]

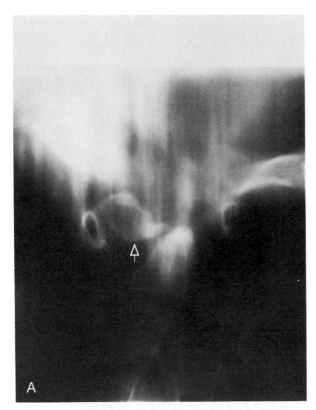

A

FIG. 5.3 Fracture of the odontoid with subluxation of the atlas on the axis. (A) Lateral pluridirectional tomogram. The fracture extends through the base of the dens (open arrow). (B) Midsagittal reformatted image demonstrating the odontoid fracture and subluxation. ·

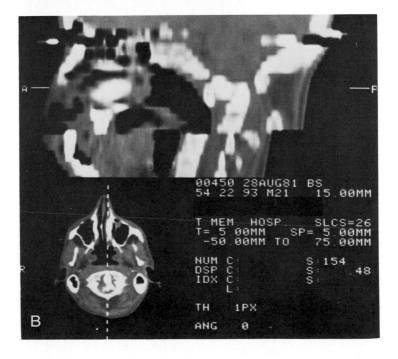

B

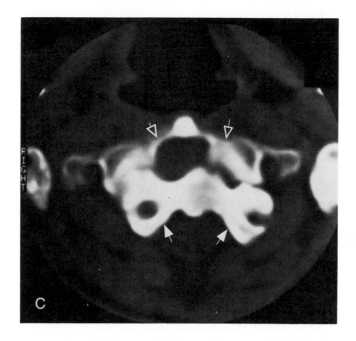

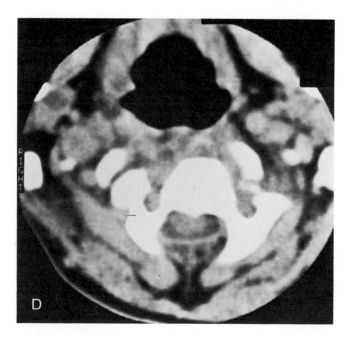

FIG. 5.3 (cont.)   (C) Axial CT section, the degree of subluxation of the atlas (open arrows) on the axis (closed arrows) is readily appreciated. (D) Compression of the anterior cervical cord by the body of the axis is also identified. Case courtesy of Dr. Victor Haughton.

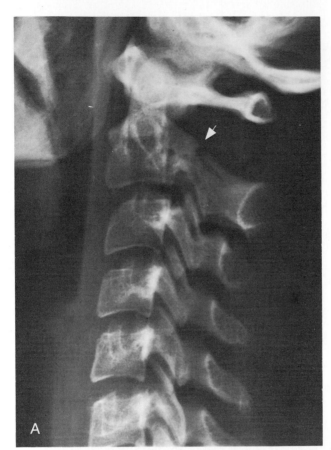

FIG. 5.4 Pseudo-hang-man's fracture. (A) Only the fracture of the lamina is identified on the plain radiograph (closed arrow).

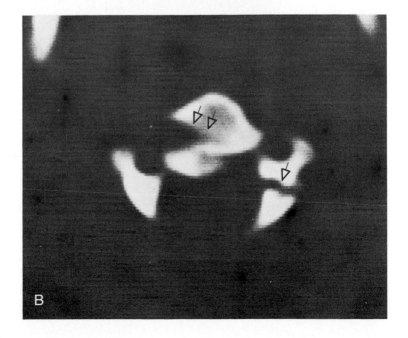

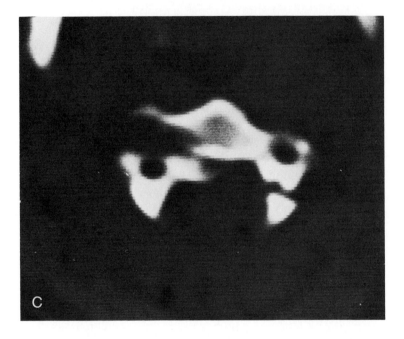

FIG. 5.4 (cont.)   (B and C) Axial CT sections reveal the complete extent of the fracture that not only involves the lamina but extends into the body of the axis (open arrows).

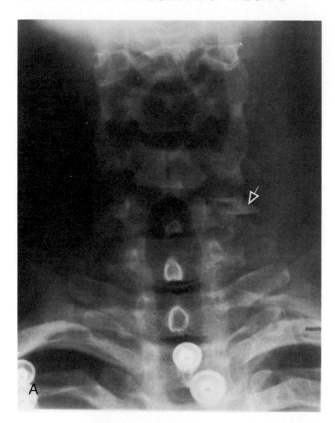

FIG. 5.5 (A) AP of the lower cervical spine with a displaced fragment of the articular pillar of C6 (open arrows). (B) In addition to the fracture involving the articular pillar there is a fracture of the lamina (closed arrows) seen on the axial CT sections.

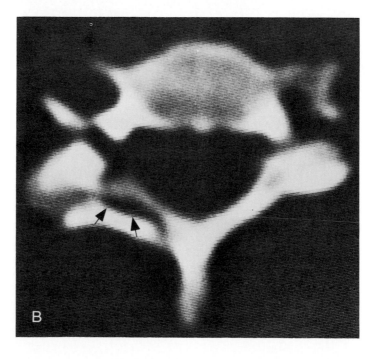

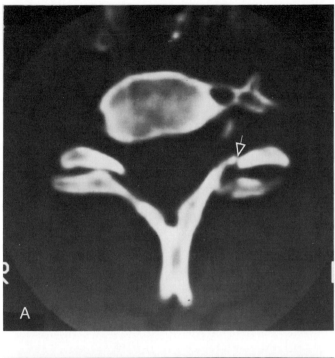

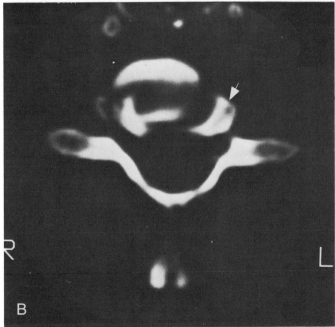

FIG. 5.6   Axial CT sections demonstrating (A) fracture through the articular pillar of C6 (open arrow) rotation of C6 and (B) probable fracture of the uncinate process of C7 (closed arrows). Case courtesy of Dr. Victor Haughton.

Hyperextension sprain (momentary dislocation) occurs when the articular and spinous processes are forced together causing rupture of the anterior longitudinal ligament and intervertebral disc.[20] CT less effectively demonstrates the decreased vertebral disc height but may be useful in identifying epidural hematoma, extruded disc material, or paravertebral soft-tissue swelling. Cautiously performed flexion extension views may be necessary to demonstrate the abnormality.[9]

Hyperextension fracture-dislocation with fracture of the articular pillar occurs when the head moves backward and downward with a component of rotation.[20] CT provides information regarding spondylolisthesis, rotation of fracture fragments, and extension of the fracture into the articular pillar.[22]

Comminuted fractures of the vertebral arch are the result of hyperextension. CT is excellent for the demonstration of fractures oriented in planes other than the transverse axial. Fractures of the spinous process, lamina, and articular pillar can usually be identified by computed tomography.

THORACOLUMBAR

Anterior compression fractures of the vertebral body are a common injury in the elderly and osteoporotic patient. These fractures are the result of flexion forces that compress and deform the vertebral body. The posterior ligamentous structures and the vertebral arch usually remain intact in interior compression fractures.

Roaf[24] has described a series of events in cadaver spines that have resulted in compression injuries. Compression forces result in bulging of the anulus fibrosus anteriorly and laterally. With increased force the end-plate fractures and a portion of the nucleus pulposus is forced through the crack into the vertebral body. Further increase in flexion results in compression of the vertebral body and if continued, disruption of the posterior ligamentous structures.

The compressive effects of spinal flexion are greatest at the anterior end of the vertebral body. The first bone injury is buckling of the anterior cortex followed by loss of vertebral body height, resulting in a wedge-shaped vertebral body. In severe injuries the intervertebral disc is torn and the nucleus pulposus may herniate in any direction. As flexion forces increase, the vertebral body is compressed and the posterior ligaments disrupted.[20]

The CT findings in anterior compression injuries include fragmentation of the vertebral end-plate and increased density of the vertebral body (zone of condensation). In addition, sagittal and coronal reformatted images permit determination of the vertebral body height (Fig. 5.7).[22]

Occasionally axial compression results in a collapse of the vertebral body resulting in a "burst" fracture. Extensive herniation of the nucleus pulposus is common. These injuries are not associated with posterior ligamentous disruption but spinal canal compromise may result from posterior displacement of fracture fragments. All compression injuries should be carefully examined to exclude facet separation or malalignment of the vertebral arches indicating instability. Computed tomography accurately assesses the severity of comminution in "burst" fractures and determines whether bony fragments have been displaced posteriorly into the spinal canal (Figs. 5.8, 5.9).[7, 25]

The spine is considered unstable when an injury permits abnormal spinal motion, which may result in neurologic deficit, deformity, or pain. Instability is usually the result of fracture of the vertebral arch, rupture of the posterior ligaments, or disruption of the facet joints. Complete destruction of the anterior structures (vertebral body and ligaments) also results in an unstable spine. The spine should be considered unstable when the CT examination reveals: 1) bilateral fractures involving the pedicles, laminae, or facet joints, and 2) when the facets no longer articulate secondary to capsular and ligamentous rupture (the "naked" facet sign). The spine is potentially unstable when there is a unilateral fracture of the pedicle, lamina, or facet joint or when there is greater than 50 percent anterior compression of the vertebral body. It must be emphasized that spine instability is a clinical diagnosis and when the injury is primarily ligamentous, the radiologic findings may be minimal.

Louis[26] has proposed a method to assess spine stability that assigns a point value to each component of injury to the vertebral column. The system of analysis focuses only on the osseous abnormalities but has been successfully applied to the evaluation of thoracolumbar injuries with CT.

Hyperflexion fracture-dislocation injuries compress the vertebral column anteriorly and distract it posteriorly. The hyperflexion force pivots around a fulcrum located in the intervertebral disc. The compression fractures are similar in appearance on CT to those described in the preceeding section.[7, 27, 28] The posterior ligamentous complex is disrupted and the vertebral arches are separated. Occasionally fractures of the pedicles and spinous processes are also present. The ligamentous injuries are not directly identifiable on computed tomography. Sagittal and coronal reformatted images allow evaluation of vertebral arch separation and fractures involving the pedicles or spinous processes (Figs. 5.10–5.12).[7]

"Seat belt"-type injuries occur when the body is hurled forward against a horizontal object. Often they are the result of sudden deceleration that occurs while the individual is wearing a seat belt. The flexion force has its fulcrum at the point of contact of the seat belt with the anterior abdominal wall. The spine lies posterior to the flexion epicenter and its components are subject to distraction forces. The vertebral column is pulled apart and compression of the vertebral body is minimal since the axis of compression is anterior in the abdominal wall.[20]

Two types of seat belt injuries are recognized. The first is a pattern in which there is a minimal compression of the vertebral body but extensive disruption of the ligamentous framework of the posterior vertebral arch with distraction of the articular processes. In these injuries the vector of force is resolved horizontally at the level of the intervertebral disc. This may be accompanied by a small compression fracture of the anterosuperior aspect of the lower vertebral body. The apophyseal joints are distracted and the intervertebral

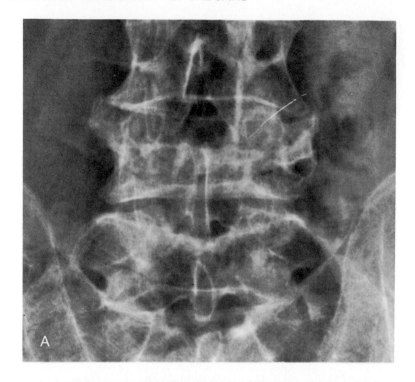

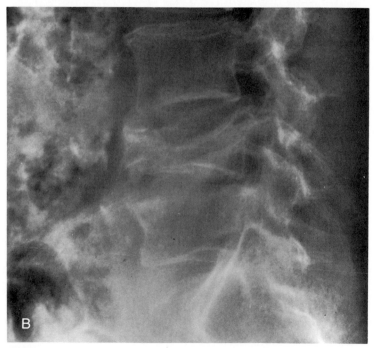

FIG. 5.7   Compression fracture of L4 in the (A) AP and (B) lateral view.

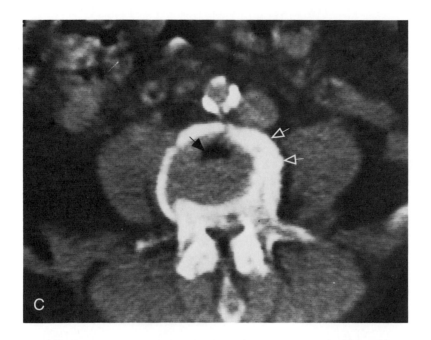

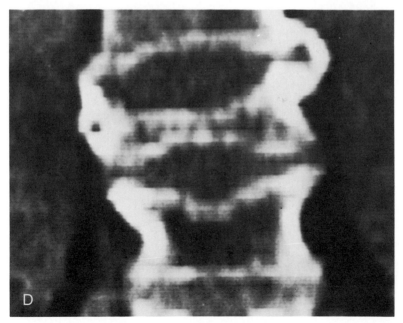

FIG. 5.7 (cont.)   (C) Axial CT section through L4 shows a region of bone condensation (open arrow) with a degenerated vacuum disc (closed arrow). (D) Coronal reformatted CT image with marked decrease in the vertebral body height.

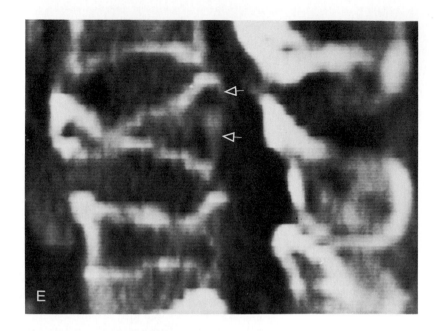

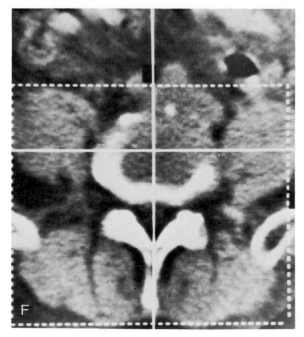

FIG. 5.7 (cont.) (E) Sagittal reformatted image with minimal posterior bulging of the vertebral body (open arrows). (F) The planes in which the reformatted images were obtained are indicated by solid white lines.

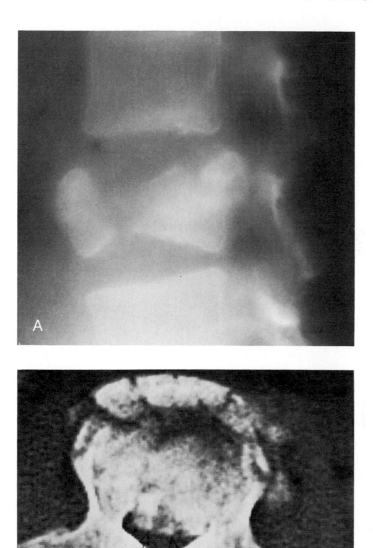

FIG. 5.8 "Burst" fracture of L2 (A) lateral pluridirectional tomogram (B) axial CT section revealing retropulsion of bony fragments into the spinal canal (open arrow).

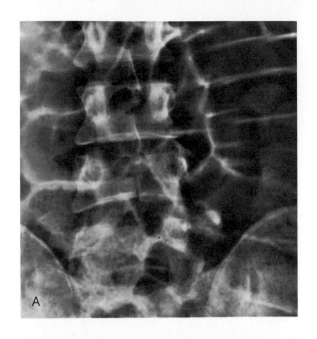

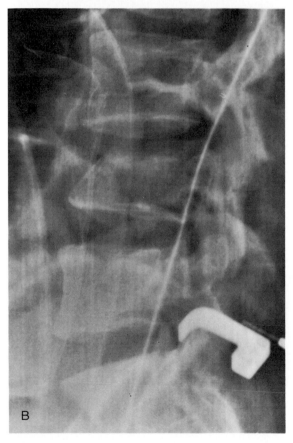

FIG. 5.9 "Burst" fracture
of L4 (A) AP and (B) lateral
radiographs.

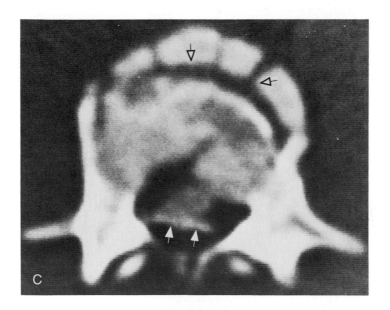

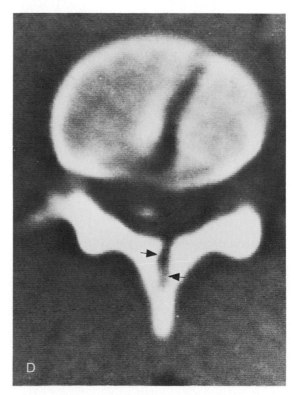

FIG. 5.9 (cont.) (C) A bone fragment is noted within the spinal canal (closed arrows) and there is a comminuted fracture of the vertebral body (open arrows). (D) CT section 5 mm more caudal demonstrating extension of the fracture into the spinous process (closed arrows).

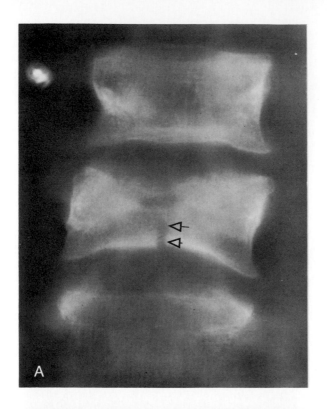

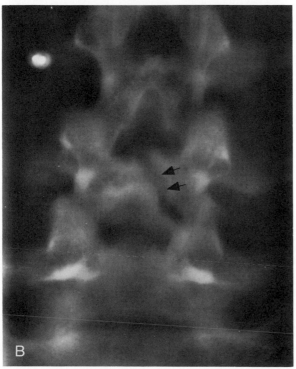

FIG. 5.10 Hyperflexion injury of L4 (A, B) AP pluridirectional tomograms demonstrate a vertically oriented fracture of the vertebral body (open arrow) with the fracture extending into the lamina (closed arrow).

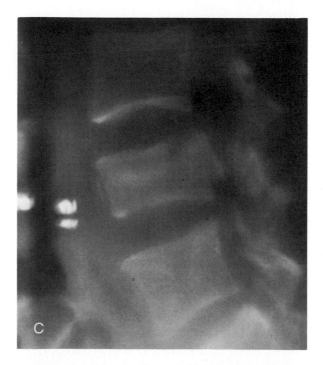

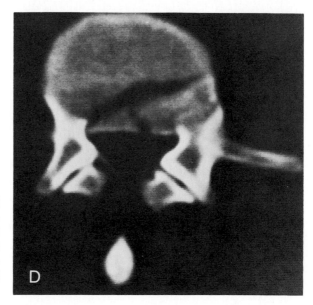

FIG. 5.10 (cont.) (C) Lateral pluridirectional tomogram revealing posteriorly displaced bony fragments. (D) The axial CT section more clearly defines the status of the spinal canal.

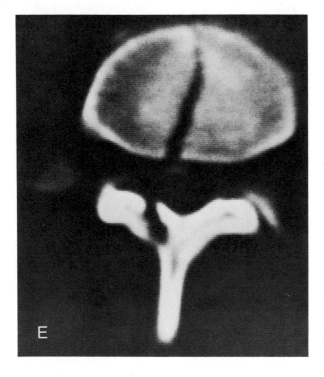

FIG. 5.10 (cont.) (E) The fracture of the lamina is also evident on the axial CT sections.

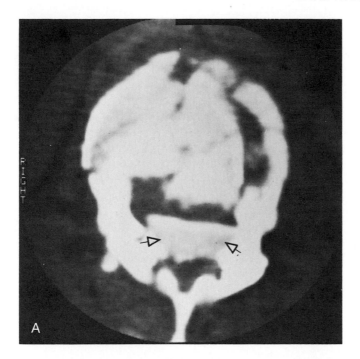

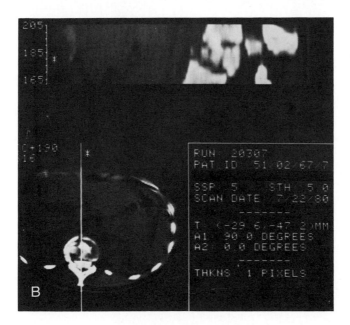

FIG. 5.11   Severe vertebral body fragmentation. (A) Axial CT scan reveals a large fragment in the spinal canal (open arrows). (B) Sagittal reformatted image allows appreciation of the separated spinous processes and identification of the intracanalicular bone fragment. Case courtesy of Dr. Victor Haughton.

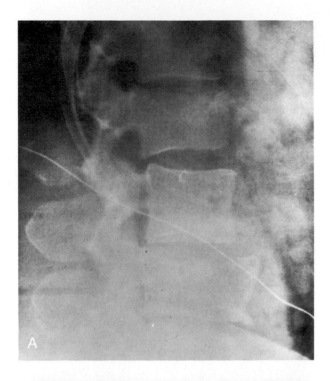

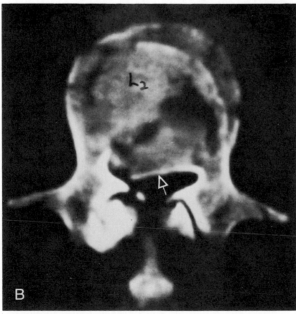

FIG. 5.12 (A) Lateral radiograph with fractures of L2 and L4 identified. (B) Axial CT section through L2 delineates the vertebral body fractures and the degree of spinal canal compromise (open arrows).

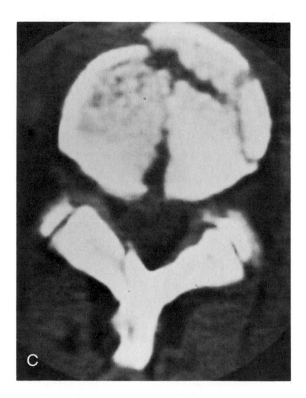

FIG. 5.12 (cont.) (C) Although there is a comminuted fracture of the vertebral body of L4 that extends into the lamina, the spinal canal is widely patent. Case courtesy of Dr. Victor Haughton.

disc is also ruptured. This vertical distraction of the articular processes is an important sign of ligamentous disruption due to flexion injuries. To demonstrate this abnormality thin transaxial CT sections must be obtained. In the region of the thoracolumbar junction, the normal apophyseal joints (superior facets, joint space, inferior facets) are visualized on a single axial section. When there is extensive posterior ligamentous disruption, the facets are distracted and the inferior facets are seen alone in the superior set of axial CT sections. The result is a "naked" facet (Fig. 5.13).[29] Subsequent scans taken at a lower level reveal the superior facets of the next vertebral level. Identification of this abnormality is clinically important in that the ligamentous injuries usually do not heal and require surgical fixation to prevent late instability. Harrington rods have been successfully utilized to achieve this goal. The second type of seat belt injury is posterior ligamentous disruption with horizontal fracture of the vertebral arch. The most commonly recognized is the Chance fracture, in which the fracture extends horizontally through the

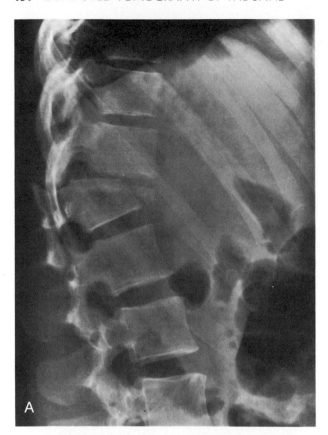

FIG. 5.13 Seat belt injury resulting in posterior ligamentous disruption and compression fracture of the vertebral body. (A) Lateral radiograph and (B,C) axial CT sections reveal that the ligamentous injury has resulted in distraction of the articulating facets.

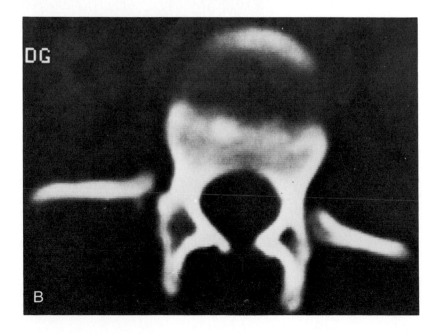

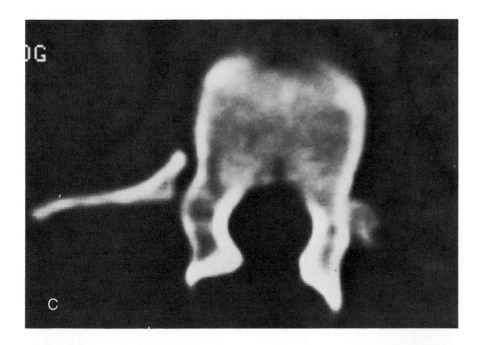

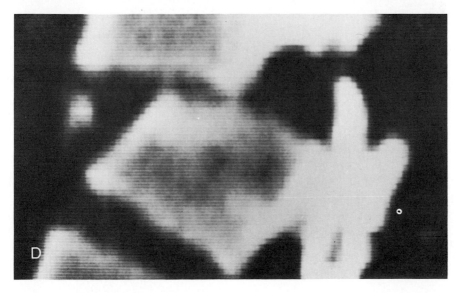

FIG. 5.13 (cont.)   On the axial CT sections, only one set of facets are visualized (the "naked" facet sign). (D) Sagittal reformatted image demonstrates anterior subluxation of T12 on L1 with the disruption of the posterior ligamentous complex.

transverse processes, lamina, pedicles, spinous process, and vertebral body.[7, 20]

Tortion forces applied to the long axis of the torso produce rotary-fracture-dislocation. There is usually associated hyperflexion. The result is disruption of the posterior ligamentous complex, which dislocates or fractures the apophyseal joints. There is a high incidence of severe neurologic deficit. Diagnosis is hampered by the tendency of the fractures to reduce themselves.

Shear fracture-dislocation occurs when there is forward force displacing the upper vertebra on the lower more stabilized vertebra (Fig. 5.14). The force is transmitted horizontally with disruption of the posterior ligamentous complex. If the vertebral arch is intact, this injury manifests itself on CT by overriding of the apophyseal joints with fracture or dislocation of the articulating processes. The anterior longitudinal ligament is torn and the vertebral body is fractured or the intervertebral disc disrupted. If the vertebral arch is frac-

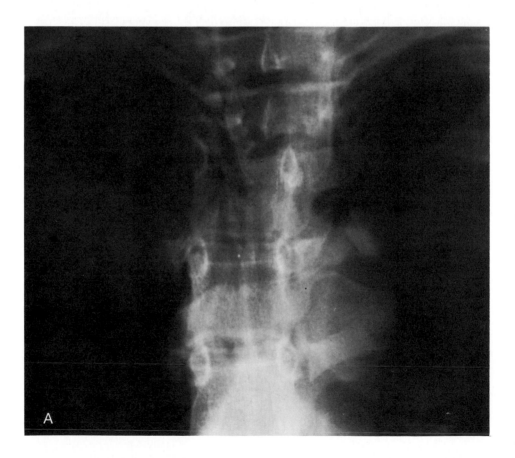

FIG. 5.14 Shear fracture-dislocation. (A) AP radiograph demonstrates severe malalignment of the upper thoracic spine.

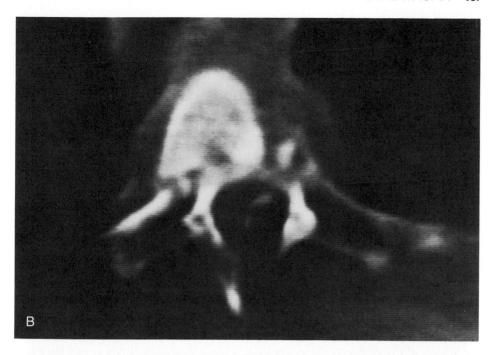

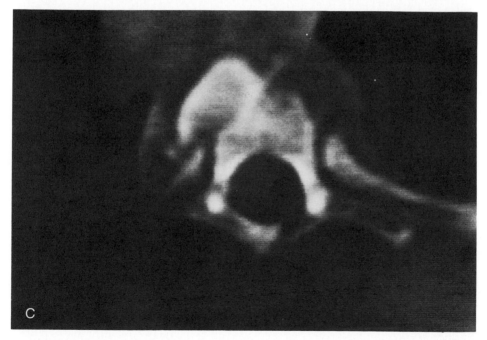

FIG. 5.14 (cont.)   (B,C) Axial CT sections reveal severe dislocation and disruption of the posterior ligamentous complex and intervertebral disc. Also noted is a paravertebral hematoma.

tured, the posterior portion of the arch and spinous process remain behind while the anterior portion moves anteriorly with the remainder of the spine.

Hyperextension fracture-dislocations are probably the result of rotation or forward shear in combination with hyperextension. There is frequent neurologic deficit. The anterior longitudinal ligament may be torn with avulsion of the disc and fracture of the posterior inferior vertebral body.

Isolated vertebral arch fractures are most often related to a direct blow to the spine. Fractures of the articular processes, transverse processes, and spinous processes have been identified with CT. Differentiation from apophyses and normal variants is important.

SACROCOCCYGEAL

CT is the ideal method to evaluate the sacrum and bony pelvis and to orient fracture fragments in relation to soft-tissue injuries. Sacral fractures are commonly produced by forces transmitted through one leg or one side of the body to the pelvis. The sacroiliac joint resists rupture and fractures occur more often along the neural foramina (Fig. 5.15). Compressive forces may be

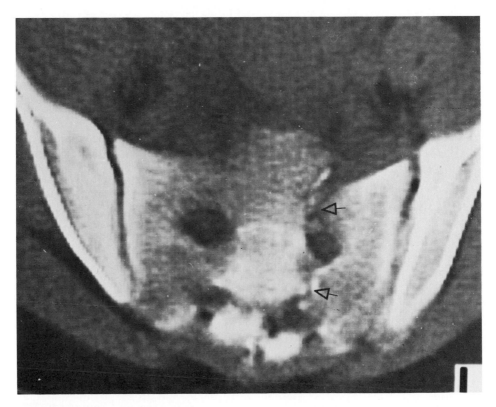

FIG. 5.15 Sacral fracture (open arrows) extending through the neural foramina.

applied to the pelvis by rotation, leverage, or shear. Leverage fractures may result in the compression of the pelvis and fracture the pubic ramus with disruption of the sacroiliac joint. Direct trauma to the sacrum may result in dislocation of the upper sacrum (Sprung Back Dislocation) occasionally associated with injury to sacral nerve roots. The coccygeal fractures are usually secondary to direct blows to the region and the pain associated with these fractures is often out of proportion to the fracture size.

PENETRATING INJURIES

Identification of foreign bodies within the spinal canal is easily accomplished with axial CT sections. The degree of fragmentation of penetrating missiles is readily determined. The location of the fragments in relationship to soft-tissue structures is also better defined than with any other radiologic modality. The relationships of foreign bodies and fracture fragments to the spinal canal are optimally demonstrated by axial CT sections.

References

1. Breasted JH: The Edwin Smith Surgical Papyrus. University of Chicago Press, Chicago, 1930.
2. Tadmor R, Davis KD, Roberson GH, New PF, Taveras JM: Computed tomographic evaluation of traumatic spinal injuries. Radiology, 127:825, 1975.
3. Colley DP, Dunsker SB: Traumatic narrowing of the dorsolumbar spinal canal demonstrated by computed tomography. Radiology, 129:95, 1978.
4. Glenn WV, Rothman SL, Rhodes ML: Computed tomography/multiplanar reformatted examinations of the lumbar spine. pp. 227–244. In Genant HK, Chefetz N, Helms CA, Eds.: Computed Tomography of the Lumbar Spine, University of California Press, Berkeley, 1982.
5. Maue-Dickson W, Trefler M, Dickson DR: Comparison of dosimetry and image quality in computed conventional tomography. Radiology, 131:509, 1979.
6. Keene JS, Goletz TH, Lilleas F, Alter AJ, Sackett JF: Diagnosis of vertebral fractures: A comparison of conventional radiography, conventional tomography, and computed axial tomography. J Bone Joint Surg, 64(A):586, 1982.
7. Brant-Zawadzki M, Jeffrey RB, Minagi H, Pitts LH: High resolution CT of thoracolumbar fractures. Am J Neuroradiol, 3:69, 1982.
8. Roub LW, Drayer BP: Spinal computed tomography: Limitations and applications. AJR, 133:267, 1979.
9. Brant-Zawadzki M, Miller EM, Federle MP: CT in the evaluation of spine trauma. AJR, 136, 1981.
10. Handel SF, Lee YY: Computed tomography of spinal fractures. Radiol Clin N Am, 19:69, 1981.
11. Powers B, Miller MD, Kramer RS, Martinez S, Gehweiler JA: Traumatic anterior atlanto-occipital dislocation. J Neurosurg, 4:12, 1979.
12. Keene GCR, Hone MR, Sage MR: Atlas fracture: Demonstration using computerized tomography. J Bone Joint Surg, 60(A):1106, 1978.
13. Fitzer PM, Nevins KF, Wendell JM: Fracture of the atlas: Demonstration by computed tomography. Virginia Medical, 106:53, 1979.

14. McInerney DP, Sage MR: Computer-assisted tomography in the assessment of cervical spine trauma. Clin Radiol, 30:203, 1979.

15. Lipson SJ, Mazur J: Anteroposterior spondyloschisis of the atlas revealed by computerized tomography scanning. J Bone Joint Surg, 60(A):1104, 1978.

16. Fielding JW, Stillwell WT, Chynn KY, Spyropoulos EC: Use of computed tomography for the diagnosis of atlanto-axial rotatory fixation. J Bone Joint Surg, 60(A):1102, 1978.

17. Rinaldi I, Mullins WJ, Delaney WF, Fitzer PM, Tornberg DN: Computerized tomographic atlanto-axial fixation. J Neurosurg, 50:115, 1979.

18. Fielding JW, Hawkins RJ: Atlanto-axial rotatory fixation. J Bone Joint Surg, 59(A):37, 1957.

19. Ghoshhajra K, Rao KCVG: CT in spinal trauma. J Comput Tomogr, 4:309, 1980.

20. Gehweiler JA, Osborne RL, Becker RF: The Radiology of Vertebral Trauma. WB Saunders, Philadelphia, 1980.

21. Haughton VM, Williams AL: Computed tomography of the spine. CV Mosby Co., St. Louis, 1982.

22. Naidich TP, Pudlowski RM, Moran CJ, Gilula LA, Murphy W, Naidich JB: Computed tomography of spinal fractures. Adv Neurol, 22:207, 1979.

23. Coin CG, Pennink M, Ahmad WD, Keranen VJ: Diving-type injury of the cervical spine: Contribution of computed tomography to management. J Comput Assist Tomogr, 3:362, 1979.

24. Roaf R: A study of the mechanics of spinal injuries. J Bone Joint Surg, 42(B):810, 1960.

25. Nykamp PW, Levy JM, Christensen F, Dunn R, Hubbard J: Computed tomography for a bursting fracture of the lumbar spine. J Bone Joint Surg, 60(A):1108, 1978.

26. Louis R: Symposium: Fractures instables du rachis tes thearies de l'instable. Rev Chir Orthop, 63:42, 1977.

27. Handelberg F, Bellemans MA, Opdecam P, Casteleyn PP: The use of computerized tomographs in the diagnosis of thoracolumbar injury. J Bone Joint Surg, 63(B):336, 1981.

28. Faerber EN, Wolpert SM, Scott RM, Belkin SC, Carter BL: Computed tomography of spinal fractures. J Comput Assist Tomogr, 3:657, 1979.

29. O'Callaghan JP, Ullrich CG, Yuan HA, Kieffer SA: CT of facet distraction in flexion injuries of the thoracolumbar spine: The "naked" facet. Am J Neuroradiol 1:97, 1980.

6 Congenital Spinal Abnormalities

JOHN P. GROGAN

To evaluate congenital anomalies including the spine and cord, the radiologist now has the choice of CT alone, with or without intrathecal enhancement, or myelography alone, or the combination of the two. The purpose of this chapter is to describe the CT appearance of the most common congenital lesions, to illustrate the advantages of myelography or CT in individual patients and to discuss logical choices of studies.

TECHNIQUE

The CT techniques chosen depend upon the congenital abnormality suspected and clinical questions to be answered. Prior to CT imaging a lateral, and sometimes an anteroposterior, localizer image is obtained to select a region of interest and plane of section. The optimal CT sections are perpendicular to rostral caudal axis of the spine. Thick slices (10 mm) and high fluxes (1100 Ma.S.) are used to obtain soft-tissue detail, especially of the spinal cord. Thin slices (1.5–5.0 mm) and moderate fluxes (500 Ma.S.) are best suited for evaluating the osseous structures. Noncontiguous sections may be used when the region of interest is extensive. Good quality reformatted images obtained with (5 or 1.5 mm), contiguous, or overlapping sections and preferably with a straight gantry have some value in selected cases.

A small dose (2–5 ml of 170 mg 1/ml) of metrizamide may be introduced intrathecally to improve visualization of the subarachnoid space, define spinal cord, and detect or confirm intramedullary and/or extramedullary cysts. Patients receiving this small amount of metrizamide experience virtually no side effects. After the contrast medium is injected into the lumbar sac, the patient may be tilted 15 degrees head down in decubitus position for 60 seconds to enhance the thoracic subarachnoid space, or for 120 seconds to enhance the cervical subarachnoid space. The C1–C2 route may also be used. CT imaging is performed with the patient supine. Metrizamide-enhanced CT may obviate the need for myelography because most of the congenital spinal abnormalities may be effectively diagnosed and demonstrated with this imaging technique. Metrizamide in the subarachnoid space permits the CT study to be performed with a very low radiation flux and a dose of one rad or less. Axial CT imaging following intravenous contrast may be useful in evaluating vascular anomalies of the cord but not dysraphism.

DIASTEMATOMYELIA

Diastematomyelia, congenital splitting of the spinal cord, may be found occasionally within a single arachnoid sheath, more commonly with separate arachnoid sheaths for each hemicord and occasionally with a fibrous cartilagenous or osseous spur separating the two cords.[29] A child with diastematomyelia may be referred for CT scanning because or radiographic demonstration of vertebral anomalies including spina bifida, widened interpediculate distance, midline bony spicule, fusion anomalies, or other abnormalities affecting a single or several segments. Or the child may be referred because of clinically observed abnormalities such as scoliosis, clubfoot, or difficulty walking with or without radiographic abnormalities.[18]

CT can demonstrate diastematomyelia as effectively as myelography.[5] If an abnormal interpediculate distance, or bony spicule or anomalous vertebral segments have been detected radiographically, this region is the one that should be studied computer tomographically. If no abnormal region of the spine has been detected, sections must be obtained at 1- or 2-cm intervals from the tip of the conus to the cervical region to exclude splitting of the cord. CT without enhancement demonstrates diastematomyelia as two distinct rounded hemicords usually within an abnormally large subarachnoid space (Fig. 6.1).[1] Each hemicord is smaller than a normal one and the two are usually unequal in size. In approximately half the cases,[41] a bony cartilaginous or fibrous structure separates the two hemicords (Fig. 6.2). In cases with an associated intramedullary cyst or hydromyelia, CT may show a low-density structure within one cord.

With metrizamide enhancement (2–5 ml of 170 mg 1/ml) and low milliamperages,[22] CT effectively demonstrates any associated meningocele and also identifies nerve roots issuing from the lateral aspect of each spinal cord. The CT examination, whether with or without metrizamide, should document the point of cord tethering.[13]

The conventional study of diastematomyelia, myelography with gas or metrizamide, is still preferred by some. When the myelogram is difficult to interpret because of confusing silhouettes or when water-soluble contrast medium concentration is considered suboptimal, CT imaging may be useful to supplement the conventional views. To have the optimal contrast medium concentration, 4 to 6 hours should elapse between myelography with metrizamide and CT imaging.

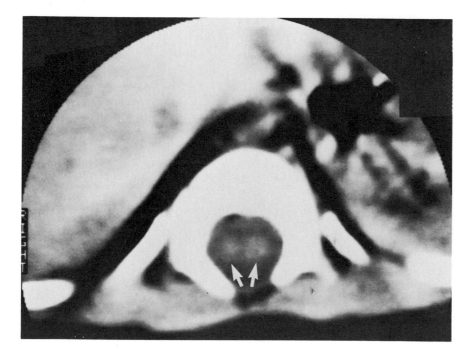

FIG. 6.1 Axial CT scan in a patient with diastematomyelia but no scoliosis, bony spur, or segmentation anomaly. The two asymmetric spinal cords (arrows) are demonstrated without any intrathecal contrast medium.

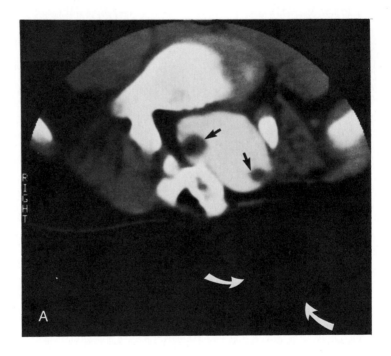

FIG. 6.2   Three axial images from a metrizamide-enhanced CT scan in a patient with diastematomyelia and a lipomeningocele. In (A) the two misshapen portions (arrows) of the spinal cord are shown within a single arachnoid sac.

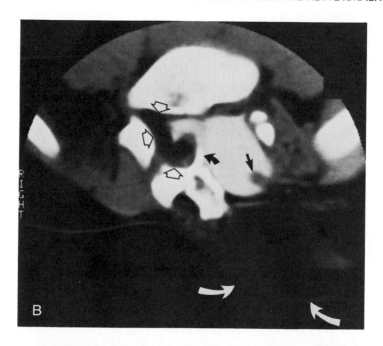

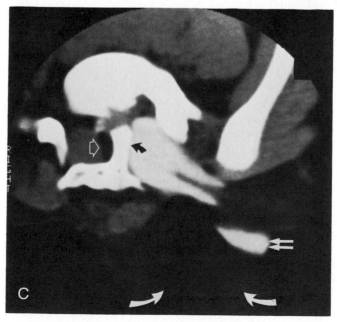

FIG. 6.2 (cont.)   (B) and (C) show the dural sac divided by a bony spur (curved black arrows). The right spinal cord ends in a small lipoma (open arrows); the left one ends in a large lipomeningocele, which fills partly with the intrathecal metrizamide (straight white arrows) and produces the soft-tissue mass (curved white arrows) on the patient's buttock.

HYDROMYELIA

Cystic dilatation of the central canal, hydromyelia, is thought to be a congenital abnormality because it occurs most frequently in association with hindbrain abnormalities.[31, 42] Unlike hydromyelia, syringomyelia is a cavitation in the spinal cord lined not by ependymal but glial cells and not always of congenital origin.[44] Syringomyelia may be idiopathic or associated with spinal cord injury, arachnoiditis, neoplasms, or degenerative conditions of the cord.[4] However, hydromyelia and syringomyelia cannot always be distinguished radiographically and therefore are discussed together.

The appearance of a syringo- or hydromyelia depends on the density and pressure of fluid within it.[14] If the cystic cavity contains fluid with a low protein concentration, CT will show the cyst as a well-defined region of low density within the spinal cord (Fig. 6.3). With higher concentrations of protein in the fluid, as with a neoplastic cyst or cavitation of the cord, the contrast

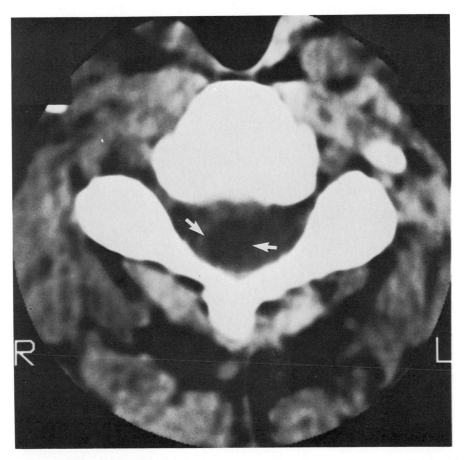

FIG. 6.3 CT demonstrating a cystic cavity (arrows) within the cervical cord. Note the sharply defined margins of the cyst.

between the cyst and the cord may be less and CT diagnosis more difficult (Fig. 6.4). If the pressure in the cyst is relatively high, the margins of the cyst are smooth, rounded, and well defined. The cyst may enlarge the cord uniformly or focally (Fig. 6.4). With tense cysts the spinal cord silhouette usually appears enlarged. When the cyst is so large that it displaces the spinal cord against the dural sac, detection of the syrinx may be difficult by CT (Fig. 6.5). If the cyst is under little pressure (flaccid cyst) it may appear small or undetectable within the cord, although the cord outline is abnormal (Fig. 6.6). As in atrophy, the dimensions of a flaccid cyst-containing cord may be abnormally small but unlike atrophy, the contour may be irregular, asymmetrical, and angular, and lack the normal oval shape (Fig. 6.7). An estimated 80 percent of spinal cord cysts can be detected by unenhanced CT.[5] Diagnostic failures are due to high protein content obscuring the cyst, misinterpretation of a spinal cord enlargement as a tumor, failure to recognize a very large cyst, or small cysts that do not deform the cord.

Metrizamide enhancement can be used to diagnose cysts not detected on routine CT imaging or to demonstrate communication of the cyst with the subarachnoid space. When cord outlines are not well visualized because of a very large intramedullary cyst, an intrathecal metrizamide-enhanced CT should be considered. In some cases metrizamide enters the cyst immediately after intrathecal injection of metrizamide; in some cases, it enters after several hours perhaps because of diffusion through the perivascular spaces[4] of the

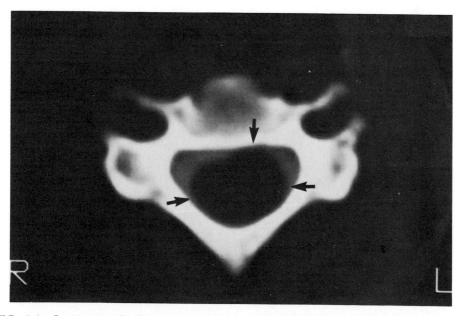

FIG. 6.4 Syringomyelia demonstrated by metrizamide enhanced CT of the cervical spine. The cord (arrows) is asymmetrically enlarged. The fluid-filled cystic cavity that was found at surgery is, however, not demonstrated by CT.

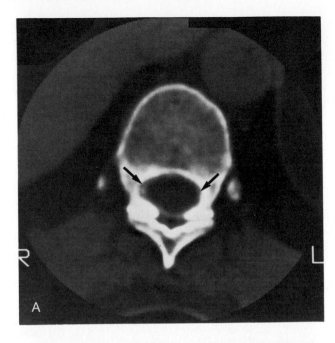

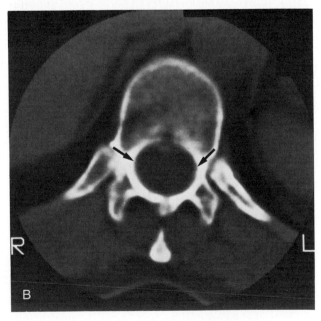

FIG. 6.5   An unusual appearance of syringomyelia in a metrizamide-enhanced CT scan. The cord silhouette is enlarged so that the subarachnoid space is thin or completely effaced (straight arrows in (A) and (B)). At surgery a syrinx was found and shunted.

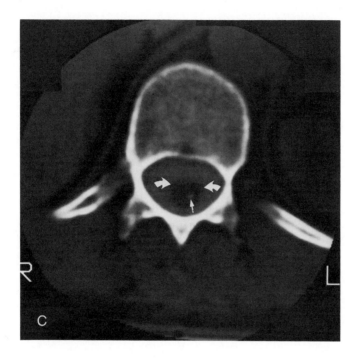

FIG. 6.5 (cont.)   A follow-up CT (C) demonstrates contraction of the spinal cord (curved arrows) and a small catheter (straight arrow) within the cavity.

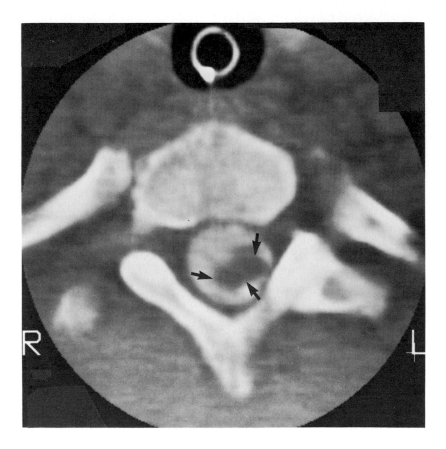

FIG. 6.6 CT demonstration of a collapsed spinal cord cyst (arrows). The spinal cord contours are irregular and abnormally small. The appearance does not suggest atrophy in which the normal elliptical shape of the spinal cord is preserved.

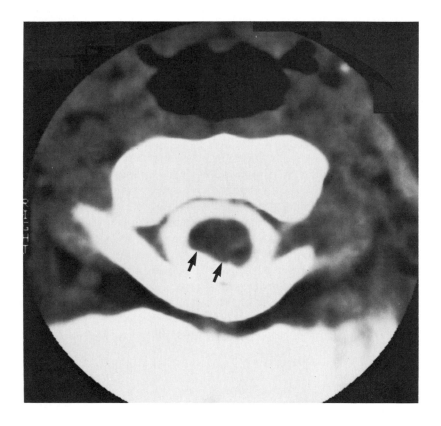

FIG. 6.7 Metrizamide-enhanced CT in syringomyelia. No definite cyst is demonstrated but the cord contour is abnormally flattened (arrows).

cord or perhaps because it communicates via the fourth ventricle;[28] in some cases metrizamide never enters a cystic space within the cord. If an unenhanced or enhanced CT scan is not diagnostic, myelography has a role in evaluating patients with suspected syringomyelia. The two-position gas myelogram is still the most effective way to demonstrate fluid movement within an intramedullary cyst.[23]

TETHERED SPINAL CORD, FILUM TERMINALE LIPOMA

A conus medullaris below the L2–L3 level in any patient older than 10 weeks is considered a tethered cord.[12]

Individuals with a tethered cord may present with an unexplained progressive urological, neurological, or orthopedic problem, may have cutaneous manifestations of spinal dysraphism such as lipomas, hypertrichosis, pigmented nevi, dermal dimples, or dermal sinuses, and may have an intradural mass (lipoma), myelomeningocele, or lipomeningocele.[26] The lipoma may be a solitary intrathecal circumscribed mass or lipomatous infiltration of the conus and/or extradural tissues. The conus itself may be normal in size despite an abnormally thickened filum terminale.[12] The dorsally situated cord may be fixed by diastematomyelia, stretched by severe scoliosis, or attached to a neural plaque in myelomeningocele or lipomeningocele.[13]

A tethered cord is most conveniently identified by myelography. While myelography can effectively identify the point of tethering and associated intradural lipomas,[19] CT may be helpful in determining extradural extension of the lipoma, lipomatous infiltration of the conus, and the demarcation between the normal cord and lipomatous tumor. Metrizamide-enhanced CT is useful in confirming the position of the conus medullaris when myelography is indeterminate and defining associated anomalies such as meningocele, neurenteric cyst, teratomatous cyst and tumors, tethering bands, and diastematomyelia.[13]

MENINGOCELE

A meningocele is a cystic dilatation of the spinal meninges. Meningocele may occur anywhere along the spinal neural axis, but most frequently in the lumbar region.

Meningocele in the cervical region occurs rarely and almost always extends posteriorly through dysraphic splayed lamina (Fig. 6.8).[30] Thoracic meningocele may be lateral or anterior. Lateral thoracic meningoceles expand through an enlarged neural foramen and then through the adjacent intercostal space to present as retropleural mediastinal masses (Fig. 6.9).[7] An anterior thoracic meningocele protrudes through a defect in the body of the thoracic vertebra into the posterior mediastinum.[38] Thoracic meningoceles must be distinguished from solid mediastinal masses.

Meningoceles in the lumbar region usually extend posteriorly beyond dysraphic posterior elements, and rarely extend laterally through several en-

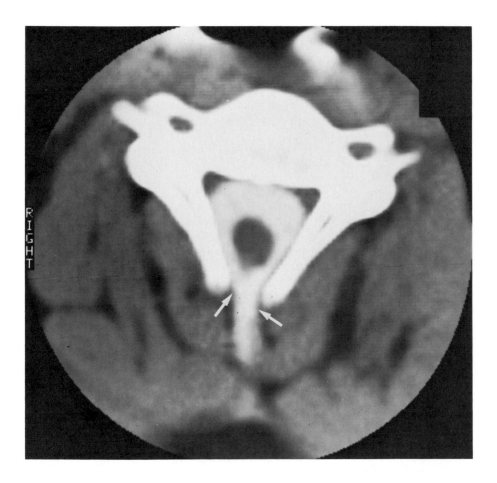

FIG. 6.8   Cervical meningocele. Metrizamide in the subarachnoid space demonstrates an abnormally shaped spinal cord and extension of the subarachnoid space (arrows) through a laminae defect. (Reproduced by permission from Haughton VM, Williams AL: Computed Tomography of the Spine, CV Mosby Co., St. Louis, 1982.)

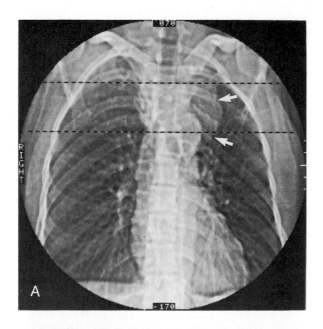

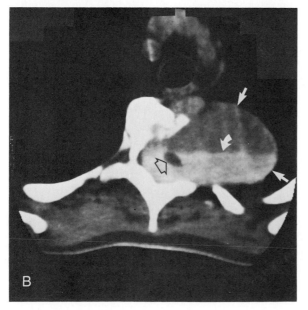

FIG. 6.9 A thoracic lateral meningocele (straight arrows) shown on the anteroposterior localizer view (A) as a mediastinal mass and confirmed to be a meningocele with axial metrizamide-enhanced CT images (B). Note the layering of the metrizamide (curved arrows) and the abnormally shaped spinal cord (open arrow). (Reproduced by permission from Haughton VM, Williams AL: Computed Tomography of the Spine. CV Mosby Co., St. Louis, 1982.)

larged lumbar neural foramina into the lumbar subcutaneous tissue and re-troperitoneum (Fig. 6.10).[10]

Sacral meningoceles may be confined to the sacrum or protrude anteriorly into the pelvis.[20] Sacral meningoceles must be distinguished from neurofi-broma, lipoma, chordoma, metastasis, and malignant neoplasms (Fig. 6.11).[17]

Meningoceles are well demonstrated on axial CT images and easily diag-nosed (Fig. 6.9). Ordinarily 5-mm-thick contiguous axial images are obtained. Larger meningoceles may be evaluated with thicker (10 mm) noncontiguous axial images. CT shows a well-defined round or elliptically shaped structure of CSF density that is contiguous with the thecal sac and extends beyond the spinal canal (Fig. 6.10). The dura is seen as a thin margin of increased density separate from the CSF. CT is useful to show the neural arch defects and define the size, location, and configuration of the meningocele.

Intrathecal metrizamide is not necessary to diagnose meningocele. It is helpful, however, in demonstrating a communication between the cyst-like structure and the dural sac. CT after intrathecal metrizamide is also helpful

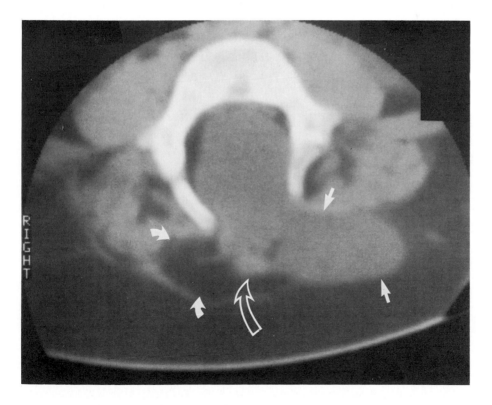

FIG. 6.10   A lumbar meningocele (straight arrows). The dural sac extends through a hiatus in the lamina. The spinal cord (large open curved arrow) and a small lipoma (small closed curved arrows) are seen.

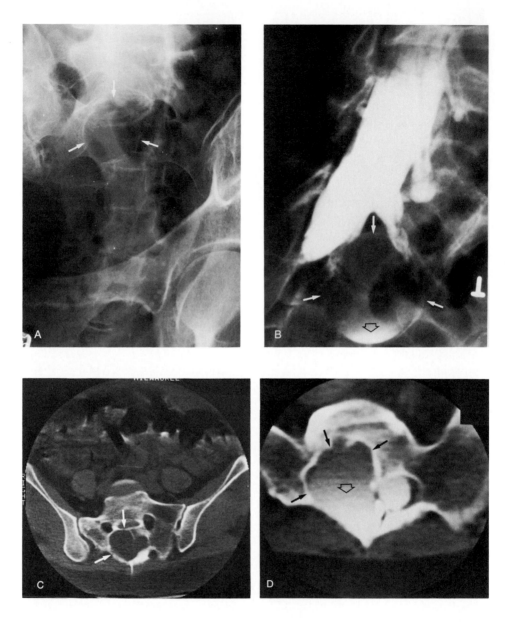

FIG. 6.11 An intrasacral meningocele. On an LAO radiograph (A), the lytic sacral defect is shown (straight arrows). RAO radiograph from a metrizamide myelogram (B) shows faint opacification (open arrows) of the cystic structure within the defect (arrows). CT images without (C) and with (D) intrathecal metrizamide confirm the presence of a meningocele (open arrow).

in identifying the location of the spinal cord relative to the meningocele. CT of myelomeningocele, a meningocele that contains neural tissue, shows neural tissue within the meningocele sac. Frequently a dorsally situated cord can be seen entering the myelomeningocele and terminating in a plaque of neural tissue (Fig. 6.2). Metrizamide-enhanced computed tomography may be helpful in detecting tethered spinal cord[19] in patients with deteriorating neurologic function following initial closure of a myelomeningocele.

ARACHNOID CYSTS

An arachnoid cyst is a diverticulum lined by arachnoid cells communicating usually with the subarachnoid space by a relatively short neck.

Arachnoid cysts may be intradural or extradural. They occur most commonly in the thoracic region and are usually located posterior to the cord and often lateral to the septum posticum. Spinal dysraphic anomalies are rarely associated with arachnoid cysts. Intradural arachnoid cysts compress, flatten, or displace the spinal cord and usually do not erode bone or enlarge the spinal canal. Extradural arachnoid cysts displace the thecal sac and usually extend through one or more intervertebral foramina and commonly erode bone or expand the spinal canal.[27] Myelography shows these intra- or extradural masses without revealing their cystic structure. Unenhanced CT usually shows the displaced spinal cord, widened spinal canal, or eroded pedicles. The arachnoid cyst cannot be resolved from the surrounding CSF with the same density. Therefore, in a patient with suspected arachnoid cyst, intrathecal metrizamide is indicated prior to CT imaging. Arachnoid cysts are seen on intrathecally enhanced CT images as well-defined, thin-walled, intradural, or extradural masses displacing and flattening the spinal cord or thecal sac (see Fig. 4.2, Chapter 4). When the CSF is enhanced with metrizamide, the arachnoid cyst remains CSF density, or increased slightly in density depending on size of the neck of the cyst and is therefore demonstrated as a filling defect in enhanced CT. Since most cysts will continue to be found initially by myelography because localization by clinical exam is difficult, CT may be considered an adjunct to myelography in the evaluation of arachnoid cysts.

NEURENTERIC CYSTS

A neurenteric cyst is an epithelium-lined structure that may occur within the spine[15] or paraspinal. The most popular theory on the development of neurenteric cysts is the persistence of the primitive neurenteric canal causing a splitting of the mesenteric canal.[6] In the cervical or upper thoracic spine, they usually enlarge the anterior subarachnoid space and flatten, compress, and displace the cord posteriorly. The cysts almost always are associated with an anterior spina bifida[33] or other congenital vertebral anomaly at the same level as the cyst. The extraspinal or paraspinal neurenteric cyst occurs most commonly in the posterior mediastinum. These cysts protruding into the right side of the mediastinum or the right hemithorax are easily recognized on chest films and must be distinguished from solid neoplasms. Mediastinal

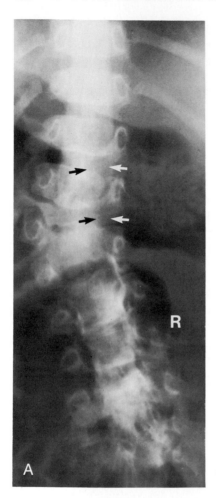

FIG. 6.12 Myelography (A) and CT (B,C) in a patient with scoliosis. Opacification of the sub-arachnoid space was suboptimal because of sco-liosis. The myelogram faintly demonstrates the spinal cord (straight arrows). The axial CT cut (B) demonstrates the abnormal position of the cord (arrowhead) and excludes tethering of the cord to the dura at this level. The reformatted coronal image

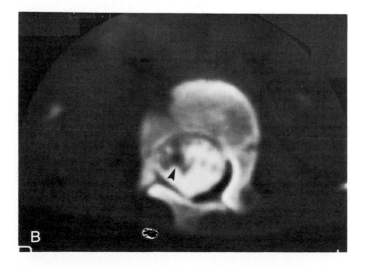

neurenteric cysts may be associated with intestinal duplication and often show adhesion or tubular communications with the meninges, spinal cord, or another intraspinal cyst.[11]

Unenhanced CT in a patient with an intraspinal neurenteric cyst will show a posteriorly displaced cord but will not usually define the intraspinal cyst since it has CSF density. Metrizamide-enhanced CT will usually outline the neurenteric cyst and the spinal cord (see Fig. 4.21, Chapter 4). The anterior location and associated dysraphic bony anomaly help to distinguish it from an arachnoid cyst, except for the isolated intraspinal epithelial cysts that may occur without a bony abnormality, which represent a variant of an enterogenous cyst.[9]

Unenhanced CT will demonstrate both the location and cystic nature of the extraspinal neurenteric cyst. Intrathecal metrizamide may be useful in demonstrating communication between the extraspinal cyst and the subarachnoid space.

SCOLIOSIS

Scoliosis may be idiopathic, secondary to structural vertebral anomalies (congenital scoliosis), or associated with neural tube defects (dysraphism).

In a scoliotic individual referred for study because of a progressive neurological deficit, the entire spinal subarachnoid space must be visualized; this is accomplished more expeditiously and with less increase in risk by metrizamide myelography than CT. In those cases of scoliosis in which myelography is suboptimal due to difficulty in moving metrizamide beyond severe scoliotic curves or dilution of contrast media, CT images should be obtained through the region of interest 4 to 6 hours following the metrizamide myelograph (Fig. 6.12). Metrizamide-enhanced CT may uncover an occult neo-

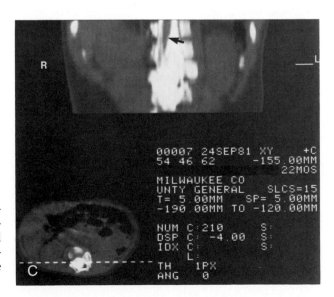

FIG. 6.12 (cont.) (C) confirms the abnormal position of the spinal cord (straight arrow). At exploration, no tethering of the cord was identified.

plasm, diastematomyelia, syringomyelia, ectopic displacement of cerebellar tonsils, spinal cord atrophy, or congenital intraspinal cyst. CT imaging after a metrizamide myelogram decreases the number of false-positive diagnoses in scoliotic children. Therefore, CT has been recommended as an adjunct to myelography in severe scoliosis, although it has less importance in mild scoliosis.[34]

DERMAL SINUS

Dermal sinus is a midline, subepidermoid cavity that connects the skin surface to a subcutaneous layer or extends into the spinal canal or cranial cavity.

Dermal sinuses most commonly occur in the lumbo-sacral region and are rare in the cervical and thoracic region. The sinus usually enters the spinal canal through dysraphic splayed lamina and the thecal sac through a defect in the dura. The sinus may attach itself to neural tissue or an intradural dermoid.

Metrizamide-enhanced CT usually demonstrates the subcutaneous tract.[40] On CT it appears as a well-defined linear collection of metrizamide extending from dorsal subarachnoid space to the surface of the skin. The sinus may be seen in continuity with a local region of cord enlargement or a dermoid. A low dose (3–5 ml) of 170 mg/ml of metrizamide is introduced into the subarachnoid space away from the site of the dermal sinus to confirm or exclude an open communication with the subarachnoid space, detect subtle cord enlargement, and identify intradural extramedullary mass (dermoid).

Acknowledgement

I would like to thank Dr. Alan Williams and Dr. David Daniels for their advice and encouragement, and Kathy M. Wutt and Debra A. Strangstalien for their secretarial assistance.

References

1. Arredondo F, Haughton VM, Hemmy DC, et al.: The computed tomographic appearance of the spinal cord in diastematomyelia. Radiology 136:685–688, 1980.
2. Balieraux-Waha D, Osteaux M, Terewinske C, et al.: The management of anterior sacral meningocele with computed tomography. Neuroradiology 14:45–56, 1977.
3. Ball MJ, Dayan AD: Pathogenesis of syringomyelia. Lancet 2:799, 1972.
4. Barnett HJM, Newcastle NG: Syringomyelia and tumors of the nervous system. In Barnett HJM, Foster JB, Hudgson P, Eds.: Syringomyelia, Major Problems in Neurology, Vol 1. WB Saunders Co., Philadelphia, 1973.
5. Bonafi A, Ethier R, Melonson D, et al.: Iligh resolution computed tomography in cervical syringomyelia. J Comput Assist Tomogr 4:42–47, 1980.
6. Bremer JL: Dorsal intestinal fistula: accessory neurenteric canal. diastematomyelia. Arch Path 54:132–138, 1952.

7. Bunner R: Lateral intrathoracic meningocele. Acta Radiol 51:1–9, 1959.

8. diChiro G, Axelbaum SP, Schellinger D, et al.: Computerized axial tomography in syringomyelia. New Engl J Med 292:13–16, 1975.

9. Fabinyi GC, Adams JE: high cervical spinal cord compression by an enterogenous cyst. Case report. J Neurosurg 51:556–559, 1979.

10. Fahrenkrug A, Hojgaard K: Multiple paravertebral lumbar meningocele. Brit J Radiol 36:574–577, 1963.

11. Fallon M. Gordon ARG, Lendrum AC: Mediastinal cyst of foregut origin associated with vertebral anomalies. Brit J Surg 41:520–533, 1954.

12. Fitz CR, Harwood-Nash DC: The tethered conus. AJR 125:515–523, 1975.

13. Fitz CR: Midline anomalies of the brain and spine. Symposium on Neuroradiology. Radiological Clin Radiol 20:95–104, 1982.

14. Gardner WJ: Hydrodynamic mechanism of syringomyelia: its relationship to myelocele. J Neural Neurosurg Psychiat 78:247–259, 1965.

15. Gimeno A, Lopez F, Figuera D, et al.: Neurenteric cyst. Neuroradiology 3:167–172, 1972.

16. Gold LHA, Kieffer SAA, Peterson HO: Lipomatous invasion of the spinal cord associated with spinal dysraphism: myelographic evaluation. AJR 107:479–485, 1969.

17. Grivegnee A, Delince P, Ectors P: Comparative aspects of occult intrasacral meningocele with conventional x-ray, myelography and CT. Neuroradiology 22:33–37, 1981.

18. Gryspeerdt GL: Myelographic assessment of occult forms of spinal dysraphism. Acta Radiol 1:702–717, 1963.

19. Heinz ER, Rosenbaum AE, Scarff TB, et al.: Tethered spinal cord following meningomyelocele repair. Radiology 131:153–160, 1979.

20. Haberbeck Modesto MA, Servadei F, Greitz T, et al.: Computed tomography for anterior sacral and intracorporal meningoceles. Neuroradiology 21:155–158, 1981.

21. Harwood-Nash DC, Fitz CR: Neuroradiology in infants and children. Vol. 3. CV Mosby Co., St. Louis, 1976.

22. Haughton VM, Williams AL: Computed Tomography of the Spine. CV Mosby Co., St. Louis, 1982.

23. Haughton VM, Williams AL, Cusick JF, et al.: A myelographic technique for cysts in the spinal canal and spinal cord. Radiology 129:717–719, 1978.

24. Healy JF, Wells MV, Carlstrom T, et al.: Lateral thoracic meningocele demonstrated by computed tomography. Comput Tomogr 4:159–163, 1980.

25. James HE, Oliff M: Computed tomography in spinal dysraphism. J Comput Assist Tomogr 1:391–397, 1977.

26. Kaplan JO, Quencer RM: The occult tethered conus syndrome in the adult. Radiology 137:387–391, 1980.

27. Kendall BE, Valentaine AR, Keis B: Spinal arachnoid cysts: clinical and radiological correlation with prognosis. Neuroradiology 22:225–234, 1982.

28. Logue V: 14th Crook–Shank Lecture. Syringomyelia: a radiodiagnostic and radiotherapeutic saga. Clin Radiol 22:2, 1971.

29. Maroun FB, Jacob JC, Hureghan WD: Diastematomyelia. Warren H Green, Inc., St. Louis, 1976.

30. Matson DD: Neurosurgery in Infancy and Childhood. 2nd ed. Charles C Thomas, Springfield, IL, 1969.

31. McRae DL: Bony abnormalities in the region of the foramen magnum: correlation of the anatomic and neurologic findings. Acta Radiol (Stockh) 40:335–354, 1953.

32. Naidich TP, McLone DG, Harwood-Nash DC: Spinal dysraphsim. In Newton TH, Potts DC Eds.: Radiology of the Skull and Brain. CV Mosby Co., St. Louis (in press, October 1982).

33. Neuhauser EBD, Harris GBC, Berrett A: Roentgenographic features of neurenteric cysts. AJR 79:235–240, 1958.

34. Petterson H, Harwood-Nash DC, Fitz CR, et al.: Conventional metrizamide myelography and computed tomographic metrizamide myelography in scoliosis. Radiology 142:111–114, 1982.

35. Raja IA, Hankinson J: Congenital spinal arachnoid cysts. Report of two cases and review of the literature. J Neurol Neurosurg Psychiat 33:105–110, 1970.

36. Resjo IM, Harwood Nash DC, Fitz CR, et al.: Computed tomographic metrizamide myelography in spinal dysraphism in infants and children. J Comput Assist Tomogr 5:549–558, 1978.

37. Resjo IM, Harwood-Nash DC, Fitz CR, et al.: Computed tomographic metrizamide myelography in syringohydromyelia. Radiology 131:405–407, 1979.

38. Rubin S, Stratemeier EG: Intrathoracic meningocele, A case report. Radiology 58:552–555, 1952.

39. Seaman WB, Schwartz HG: Diastematomyelia in adults. Radiology 70:962–965, 1958.

40. Scotti G, Harwood-Nash DC, Hoffman HS: Congenital thoracic dermal sinus: Diagnosis by computer assisted metrizamide myelography. J Comput Assist Tomogr 4:675–677, 1980.

41. Scotti G, Musgrave MA, Harwood-Nash DC, et al.: Diastematomyelia in children: Metrizamide and CT metrizamide myelography. AJR 135:1225–1232, 1980.

42. Spillane JD, Pallis D, Jones AM: Developmental abnormalities of the foramen magnum. Brain 80:11–48, 1957.

43. Weinstein MA, Rothner AD, DuChesneau P, et al.: Computer tomography in diastematomyelia. Radiology 118:609–611, 1975.

44. Williams B: Pathogenesis of syringomyelia. Lancet 2:969–970, 1977.

45. Wolpert SM, et al.: Computed tomography in spinal dysraphism. Surg Neurol 8:199–206, 1977.

7 Spondylolysis

VICTOR M. HAUGHTON

Spondylolysis is defined as a defect in the pars interarticularis. Whether it is congenital or acquired, symptomatic or incidental, however, is debated in many cases. The problem spondylolysis poses for CT interpretation is that the defect may simulate a facet joint and therefore be misinterpreted.

Spondylolysis has several characteristic CT features (Fig. 7.1). The spondylolytic defect is usually detected in a cut that intercepts the pedicles. The defect appears as a ragged interruption in the pars, oriented in a roughly verticle plane, lacking cortical margins, and usually with sclerosis of the adjacent bone. CT is likely to show an abnormally long anteroposterior diameter of the spinal canal and osseous processes that project inferiorly from the abnormal pars (Figs. 7.1, 7.2), and if spondylolisthesis is present, distortion of the posterior margin of the adjacent intervertebral disc (Fig. 7.3).

The plane of a pars defect and of the facet joint are nearly identical. Therefore in axial CT sections, a pars defect between the anterior and posterior part of the pars interarticularis may resemble the joint space between the superior and inferior articular processes (Fig. 7.4). The key to recognizing a spondylolytic defect is identifying the inferior and superior articular processes of a vertebra. A space separating parts of adjacent vertebrae is an articulation; a defect within one vertebral pars is a spondylolysis. The facet joints, which are described in detail in Chapter 1, can also be distinguished from spondylolysis by other features, for example, the even uniform articular cortical surfaces, the uniform space separating bone, the notch adjacent to the inferior process, which characterize facet joints but not spondylolysis. Since the facet joints near a spondylolysis rarely degenerate, the sclerosis and irregularity near a spondylolysis distinguish it from the adjacent joints. In many cases the pars defect can also be confirmed by examining the localizer image. In more difficult cases, reconstructed images or conventional radiographs will confirm the diagnosis.

The pars abnormalities may have a number of bizarre appearances (Fig. 7.5). Although the spondylolysis is commonly bilateral, the unilateral ones can be recognized, often with considerable sclerosis in the contralateral at

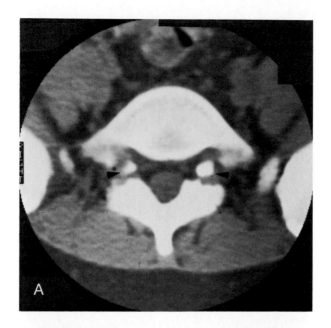

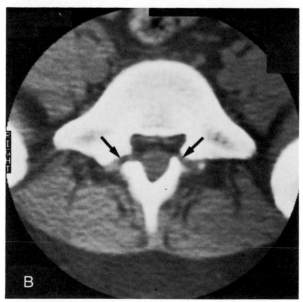

FIG. 7.1 Atypical appearance of spondylolysis in axial CT scans. The two contiguous 5-mm thick slices show the bilateral pars defects (arrows) in L5, sclerosis and irregularity of the adjacent margins of the defect, prominent osseous processes (arrowheads) just beneath and anterior to the pars defects, and the elongation of the spinal canal.

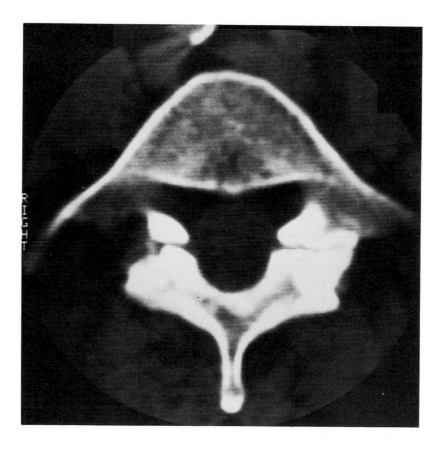

FIG. 7.2   The hyperostosis and sclerosis adjacent to spondylolysis. The cortical margins adjacent to the spondylolysis are thickened at the expense of the medullary cavity on either side.

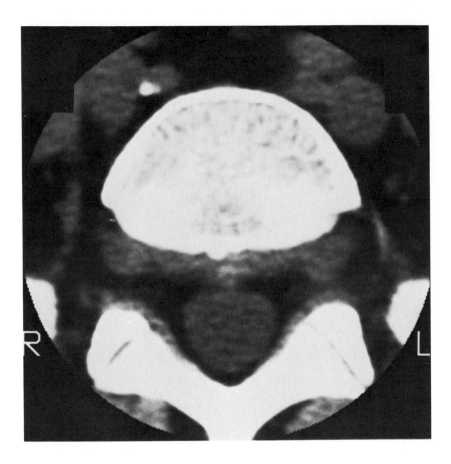

FIG. 7.3   The posterior margin of the L5–S1 disc in a patient with an L5 spondylolysis and spondylolisthesis. Note that the disc appears to protrude symmetrically beyond the L5 vertebra. The ganglion (arrows) appear to be contiguous to the disc margin.

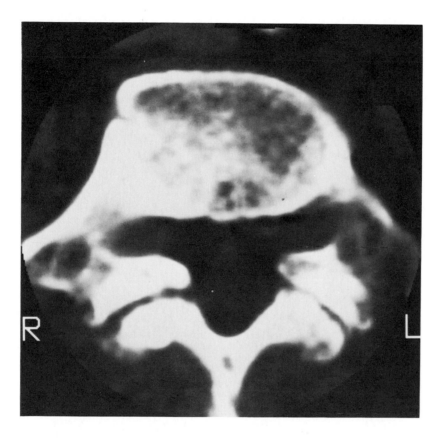

FIG. 7.4 The slice through the pars of L5 shows structures resembling a facet joint. However, all the bone present is part of the L5 vertebral body. The spaces are pars defects not joints (confirmed radiographically and surgically). The sclerosis and irregularity are not typical of facet joints, which in this patient had some very minor degenerative changes.

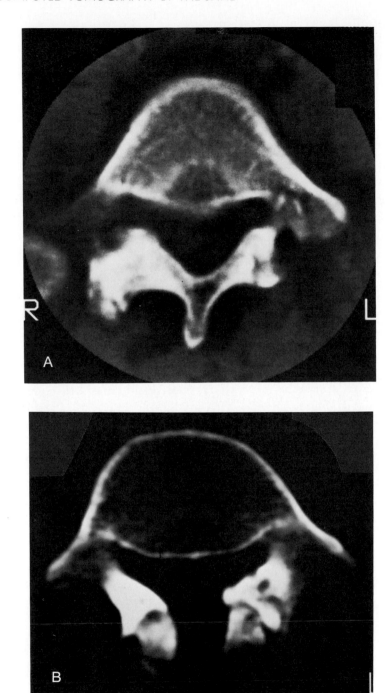

FIG. 7.5 Unusual examples of spondylolysis. (A) Predominantly unilateral sclerosis of the pars. (B) spondylolysis and cystic changes in the pars bilaterally.

pars interarticularis (Fig. 7.5A).[4] In some cases, the pars appears abnormally thin and elongated with (Fig. 7.5B) or without a disc continuity in the pars (Fig. 7.6).[3] In some cases sclerosis in the pars can be identified without a discontinuity.[3] The relationship of these abnormalities in the pars interarticularis to the common form of spondylolysis and to clinical symptomatology must be investigated further.

The accuracy of CT versus plain radiographs in identifying spondylolysis has not been studied. Although the diagnosis of spondylolysis by conventional radiographs is usually reliable, defects may be obscured in some projections because of overlying silhouettes or because of myelographic contrast media present in root sheaths. Therefore, some examples of pars articularis defects overlooked by conventional films but demonstrated by CT have been collected.[1] Examples of spondylolysis missed by CT, especially when the defect resembles the facet joints, may also be noted.[3]

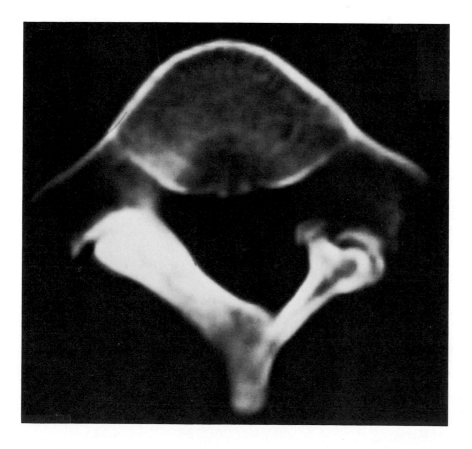

FIG. 7.6. In this patient a unilateral pars defect is present on the left and sclerosis of the pars on the right. A hypoplastic left superior articular process of S1 can be seen. This case illustrates the association of anomalous facet joints and spondylolysis.

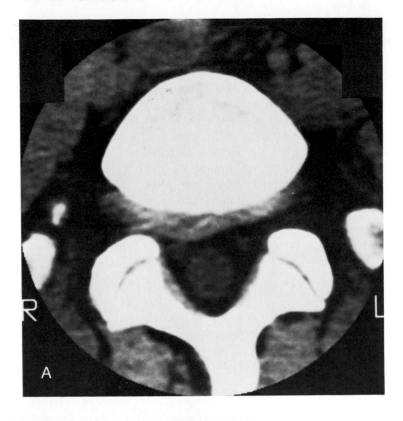

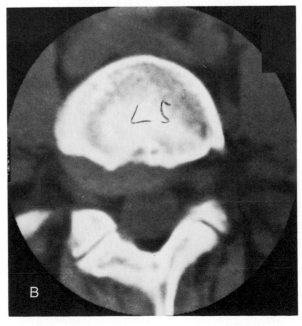

FIG. 7.7 Herniated disc and spondylolysis. (A) A spondylolysis and spondylolisthesis distort the posterior disc margin. A nuclear herniation causes the asymmetry. Note that the S1 root sheath is displaced posteriorly. Myelography confirmed the radicular compression (see Ch. 7). (B) The posterior disc margin appears asymmetric but note that the cut intercepts the disc margin obliquely. The asymmetry is technical in origin not due to a herniation. Note also that fat separates the L5 spinal nerves from the posterior margin of the disc in this particular case.

Distortion of the posterior margin of the intervertebral disc is a characteristic of spondylolysis complicated by spondylolisthesis. The problem with this distorted disc margin is to distinguish it from a herniated disc associated with spondylolysis.[2] The distortion of the posterior disc margin due to spondylolysis is usually symmetrical (Fig. 7.3) unless scoliosis is present or cuts intercept the spine at an angle. A disc herniation produces an asymmetric posterior disc margin (Fig. 7.7). A herniation, therefore, can be suspected when the disc margin appears to protrude asymmetrically without a technical explanation for the asymmetry and can be substantiated by finding evidence on the CT images of nerve root compression (See Chapter 2). Displacement of the root sheath or obscuring of a spinal nerve within the spinal canal suggests that a herniation is present. When fat can be demonstrated around the spinal nerves and root sheaths, herniation should probably not be diagnosed. In some cases myelography may be necessary for confirmation or exclusion of a herniated disc.

References

1. Haughton VM, Eldevik OP, Magnaes B, Amundson P: A prospective comparison of computed tomography and myelography in the diagnosis of herniated lumbar disks. Radiology 142:103–110, January 1982.
2. Eldevik OP, Dugstad G, Orrison WW, Haughton VM: The effect of clinical bias on the interpretation of myelography and spinal CT. Radiology 145:85–90, 1982.
3. Grogan J, Hemminghytt S, Daniels D, Williams AL, Haughton VM: Spondylolysis studied with computed tomography. Radiology 145:737–742, 1982.
4. Sherman FC, Wilkinson RH, Hall JE: The reactive sclerosis of a pedicle and spondylolysis in the lumbar spine AB. Radiology 124:571, 1977.

8 The Role of CT Scanning in Spinal Surgery—A Surgeon's Perspective

PATRICK R. WALSH

The advent of computed tomographic (CT) techniques has been hailed as the dawn of a new era in neuraxial imaging. In reflection of convenience, safety, and sensitivity, CT scanning has assumed a position of almost undisputed value in the management of a wide range of neoplastic, infectious, demyelinating, and hemorrhagic cranio-cerebral disease processes. Sophisticated segmental localizing features, larger gantry apertures, and improved resolution have led to the enthusiastic application of CT imaging to the spinal segment of the neuraxis. Advantages of CT over previously available spinal roentgenologic techniques have become apparent in the relatively brief period of high-resolution scanner availability.[11, 35] This chapter seeks to address the impact of CT scanning on surgery of the spinal column, cord, and nerve roots.

Surgical and related neuroradiologic considerations commence with clinical data, which in the setting of spinal disease processes most frequently include historical, physical, and possible electrodiagnostic (electromyography and somatosensory-evoked potentials[15]) evidence of myelopathy or radiculopathy. The temporal course of the process and features of pain are frequently of value in etiologic definition. Rational surgical planning presupposes precise appreciation of the extent and nature of responsible anatomic osseous, neural, or soft-tissue lesions. CT scanning has been shown to be highly sensitive in depiction of detail of this type,[11, 14] and such data have been employed to create a schema for surgical planning in lumbar spondylosis,[22] disc disease,[1] and spinal fracture.[6, 25] In addition surgical planning requires appreciation of spinal columnar instability, extant or potential, which may develop differentially upon exposure to transient or plastic (static-deforming) forces.[19, 23] Instability may be inferred from radiographically demonstrated static abnormalities, including fractures and osseous displacements, to which CT scanning is sensitive; however, acute instability is a dynamic process. Definitive proof of stability may require roentgenologic evaluation during cautious, transient force application through flexion–extension or other stressed films of the spinal column. Displacements of dural or ligamentous structures may distort the neural elements in the absence of obvious spinal instability[2, 26] and elicit symptomatology;[15] demonstration of such perturbations by CT scanning requires careful attention to patient position and scanning planes.

As the title of this chapter indicates, this section should be viewed as *a* surgeon's perspective. Although an attempt to address general issues will be forthcoming, variability of imaging preferences exists among surgeons and among neuroradiologists. The ideal spinal neuroradiologic technique would image and localize neural, osseous, and soft-tissue components of the spinal column at minimal patient risk and morbidity with maximal sensitivity and precision. At issue is the ability of CT scanning to approach these goals and to disclose supplemental information not obtainable by myelography or routine radiographs and therein to improve the focus of surgical planning. Critical evaluation of the potential contributions of spinal CT scanning requires an appreciation of the relative roles of conventional roentgenologic techniques. The risks associated with lumbar puncture and contrast agents have been documented,[10, 21, 28, 34] and a number of surgeons have opposed the routine use of myelography in evaluation of radiculopathy. These surgeons cite the frequency of myelographic abnormalities in asymptomatic patients and the 25 percent "false-negative" rate[8, 9, 13, 24] of myelography and maintain that the diagnosis of radiculopathy is more firmly established on clinical than radiologic evidence.[17, 27] In this setting, spinal CT scanning represents a revolutionary advance that permits anatomic spinal evaluation without the risks that attend myelography. A probably larger group of surgeons routinely employ myelography in the evaluation of disc disease; for this group, CT imaging may provide either an alternative or supplement to myelography.

The utility of CT scanning in definition of the anatomic perturbations of spinal trauma, neoplasm, disc disease, and congenital processes, as well as of intrinsic abnormalities of the spinal cord, has constituted the focus of attention of a number of contributors to this edition. Consequently, only selected cases in which CT was of value in surgical management will be presented. The first disease category to be reviewed will be neoplasia. Figures 8.1 and 8.2 illustrate neurofibromata in the upper cervical spine that were well delineated by CT scanning. Extraforaminal tumor extension directs surgical scope beyond simple laminectomy and was precisely defined only by CT scanning. Figures 8.3 and 8.4 illustrate additional cases in which data of surgical import, which could not be obtained from myelography, were derived from CT scanning. In Figure 8.3, presacral and prevertebral metastatic tumor may be seen to involve the region of the lumbar plexus in the absence of myelographically defined neural distortion. In another patient with prostatic cancer and myelopathy, combined air-metrizamide myelography demonstrated complete block, related to epidural metastasis (Fig. 8.4), but did not delineate the radial distribution of tumor within the canal; this infor-

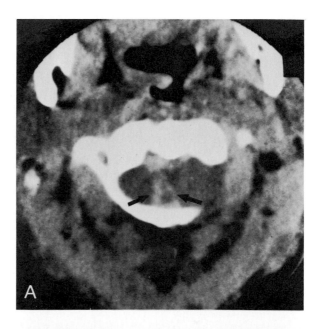

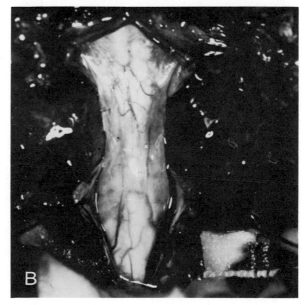

FIG. 8.1   C1–2 bilateral neurofibromata. (A) Note marked
distortion   of   metrizamide
enhanced dural sac (arrows)
and cervical spinal cord by
bilateral low-density neurofibromata without major extraforaminal extension. (B)
Operative photograph after
C1–C2   laminectomy   and
complete resection of bilateral
extradural   neurofibromata
that did not require extraforaminal dissection.

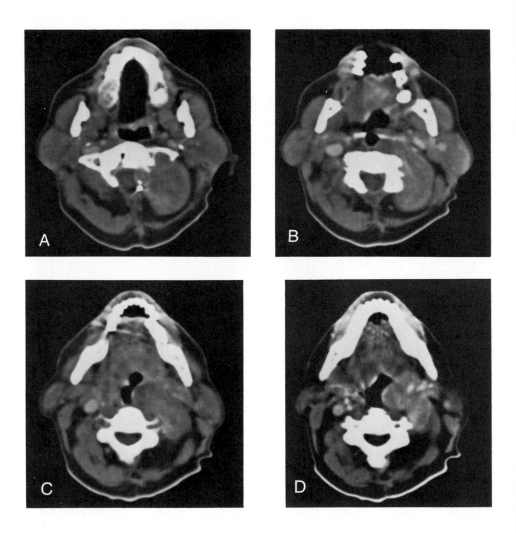

FIG. 8.2 Cervical neurofibroma. In contrast to the patient in Figure 8.1, massive extraforaminal tumor extension is evident. Observe distortion of neural elements and massive extraforaminal tumor extension to muscular and pharyngeal sites. (A–D successive cranial to caudal continuous sections.)

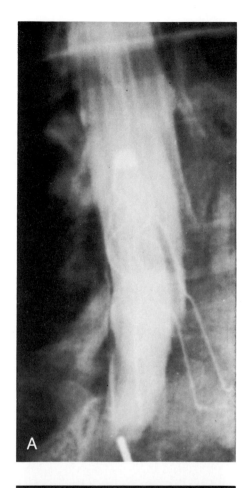

FIG. 8.3 Retroperitoneal metastasis. (A) Metrizamide lumbar myelogram in patient with profound lower extremity paresis. Abdominal surgical clips and caval interruption device are noted with minimal myelographic abnormality. CT sections (B,C) demonstrate sacral erosion and prevertebral tumor mass with probable infiltration of lumbar plexus and involvement of the L5 vertebral body.

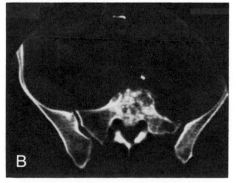

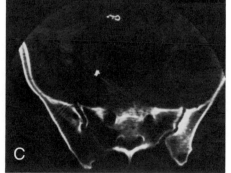

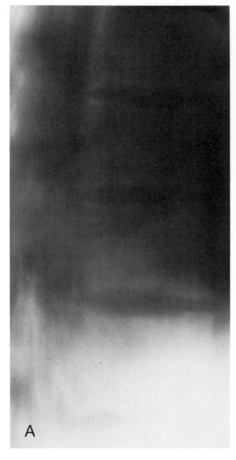

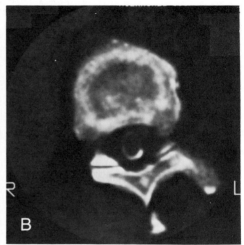

FIG. 8.4 Epidural metastasis. (A) Polytomographic image of myelogram obtained after cervical injection of oxygen and lumbar injection of metrizamide demonstrates complete block, but does not define radial disposition of tumor bulk within the canal. (B) CT image demonstrates increased anteroposterior diameter of the spinal cord and bilateral lateral tumor confirmed at surgery.

mation, coupled with knowledge of vertebral body status, is of major importance in determination of surgical approach to such lesions (laminectomy versus anterior or lateral decompression). Bilateral laterally situated tumor bulk, distorting the spinal cord and subarachnoid space, was demonstrated by metrizamide-enhanced CT and was confirmed at surgery. An unusual extradural compressive mass, hypertrophic extradural fat, accompanying high-dose steriod administration after renal transplantation, is to be seen in Figure 8.5; although conventional myelography may demonstrate related

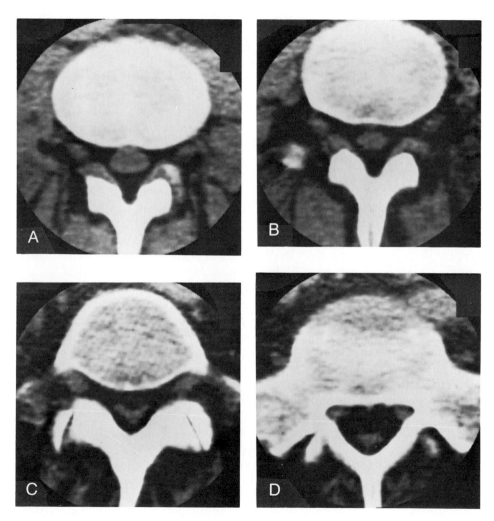

FIG. 8.5   Hypertrophy of lumbar epidural fat due to high dose steroid immunosuppression after renal transplantation with lumbar stenotic canal syndrome. Note increased prominence of epidural fat and progressive narrowing of the lumbar theca at caudal levels (A,L3; B,L4; C and D, L5–S1).

stenosis of the lumbar theca, the nature of this epidural tissue is most precisely defined through the sensitivity of CT to tissue density differences.

CT scanning may also be a valuable supplement to myelography in non-neoplastic disease processes, especially with anatomic perturbations situated lateral to the myelographically visualized nerve root sheaths[16] (Figs. 8.6, 8.7). Laminotomy without foraminal exploration in cases such as these fails to identify or relieve radicular compression and may be responsible for a number of so called "failed back" syndromes. Sciatica with relatively little lumbar pain is a common presentation of lateral compressive syndromes, and patients frequently experience exacerbation of symptoms with lumbar extension rather than straight-leg raising. Relative absence of lumbar pain in these patients presumably reflects radicular compression distal to recurrent spinal branches; the etiology of lower-extremity pain has been intensely debated as both ischemic and direct axonal compressive hypotheses have been forwarded. A calcific component of disc herniation may suggest modification of surgical technique through extension of dorsal elemental resection and curettage; such calcification is often clearly demonstrated by CT scanning (Figs. 8.7 and 8.8). Aggravation of pain by extension may reflect dynamic foraminal stenosis through infolding of the dura or ligamenta flava;[26] hypertrophy of this ligament is apparent in Figure 8.9. A synovial cyst (Fig. 8.10) may occasionally elicit similar dynamic stenosis. Nervous tissue behaves as a liquid of constant volume, and Brieg has demonstrated an increase in the diameters of neural elements with extension associated shortening;[2] enlargement of neural elements in a marginal canal or foramen, further narrowed by extension, may transiently augment stenosis and is likely a factor in the development of neurogenic claudication[31, 36] and postural symptomatology.[33] Neurogenic claudication was a complaint common to patients illustrated in Figures 8.11 through 8.14; in each of these patients static lumbar stenosis was present. Spinal stenosis has been divided into generalized, localized, and segmental forms, due to either congenital or spondylotic processes.[7, 20, 29, 30, 32, 37] Achondroplasia provides the prototype of congenital spinal stenosis, characterized by pedicular shortening with resultant reduction of all canal sagittal diameters. Canal compromise arises from a posterolateral vector with degenerative-acquired or spondylitic spinal stenosis on the basis of facet and ligamentous hypertrophy and disc protrusion in varying combinations. In Figure 8.11 the configuration of the spinal canal demonstrates elements of both congenital and spondylotic stenotic processes at different levels. In Figure 8.11 enlargement of facets produced severe foraminal stenosis, whereas, in Figure 8.12, a similar process primarily affected the canal and lateral recesses. The importance of scanning multiple levels is apparent upon review of Figure 8.13; canal diameters are minimally reduced at low lumbar segments, however, profound stenosis is in evidence at the L2–L3 interspace. The obligate segmental focus of CT scanning dictates scanning of multiple levels in the setting of presumed stenosis and consideration of myelography to evaluate extended segments of the neuraxis. CT may be of special value in segmental evaluation not provided by myelography in patients in whom

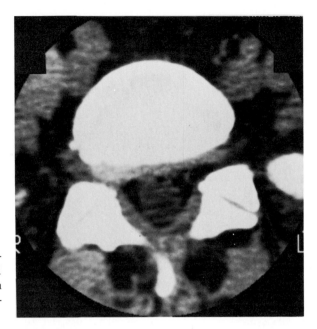

FIG. 8.6 Far lateral (foraminal) disc prolapse at L5–S1 with associated calcification with clinical lateral disc syndrome.

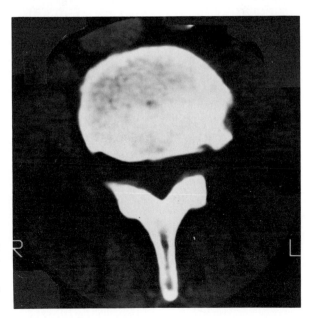

FIG. 8.7 Extraforaminal disc prolapse with associated osteophytic formation at L4–L5. Note left L4 radicular displacement.

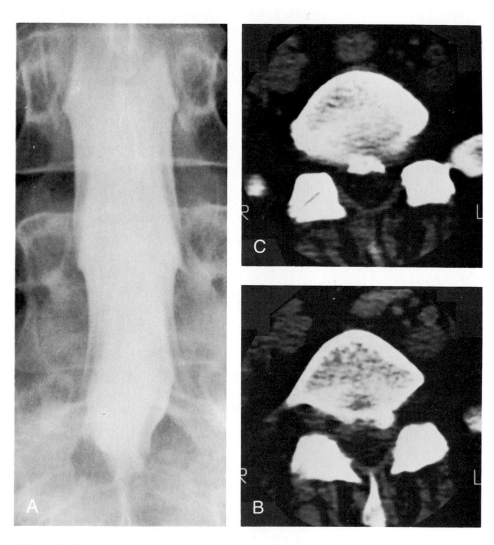

FIG. 8.8 Unilateral sciatica. (A) Metrizamide myelographic image demonstrates left extradural defect at L5–S1. (B) CT image from cephalic L5–S1 interspace demonstrates calcific component of the disc prolapse not apparent on myelography. (C) Image obtained slightly caudal to B demonstrates extensive soft-tissue mass with obliteration of epidural fat and further foraminal compromise.

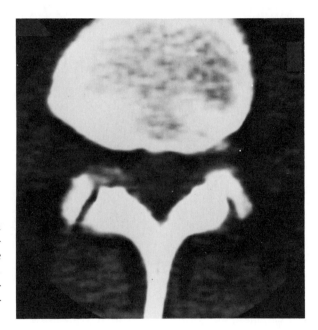

FIG. 8.9   CT scan at L4–L5 in patient with sciatica and minimal lumbar pain compatible with foraminal syndrome. Note prominence of ligamentum flavum at facet with compromise of foramen.

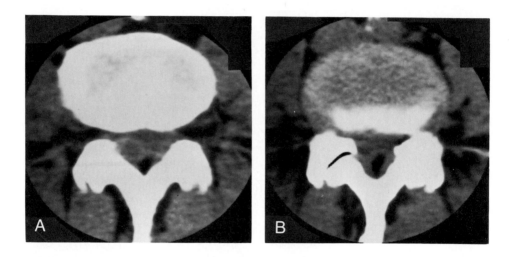

FIG. 8.10   Sciatica with minimal lumbar pain compatible with foraminal syndrome. (A) Note spherical circumscribed mass extending ventromedially from region of right L4–L5 facet suggestive of synovial cyst. (B) Repeat image obtained 7 weeks later, by which time the patient had achieved dramatic symptomatic relief. Note reduction in size of mass.

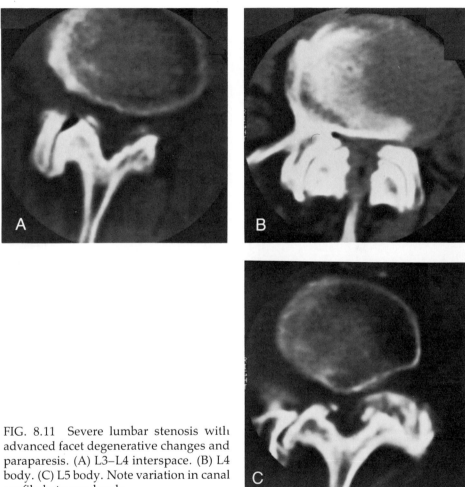

FIG. 8.11 Severe lumbar stenosis with advanced facet degenerative changes and paraparesis. (A) L3–L4 interspace. (B) L4 body. (C) L5 body. Note variation in canal profile between levels.

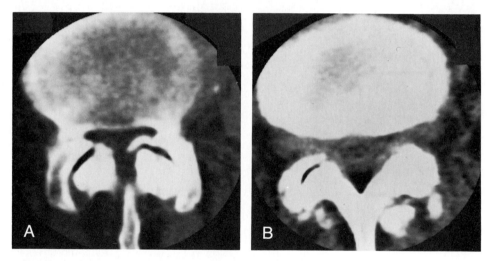

FIG. 8.12 CT in neurogenic claudication with paraparesis and postural aggravation of pain. (A) L3–L4 interspace. Observe severe stenosis of lateral recess and lateral constriction of lumbar theca secondary to facet degenerative changes with marked ventromedial migration of left superior articulating process. (B) Similar but much less severe changes at L4–L5.

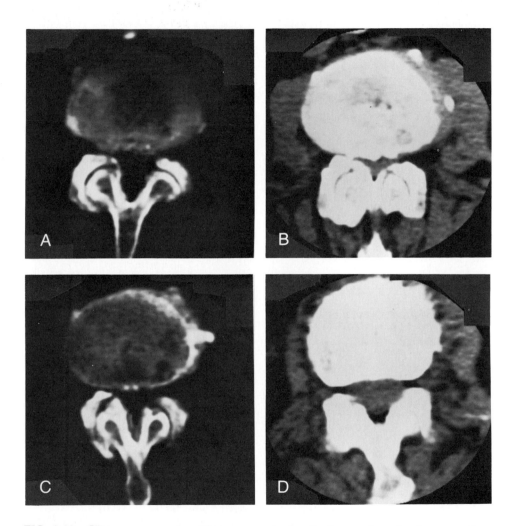

FIG. 8.13   CT in paraparesis with neurogenic claudication and postural aggravation of pain with sphincteric dysfunction and upper lumbar stenosis. (A) Upper L4 body. Observe severe right foraminal stenosis with osteophytic formation and facet enlargement. (B) Profound stenosis at superior edge of L2–L3 interspace with marked reduction of anteroposterior canal diameter in addition to foraminal narrowing. (C) Observe more triangular canal format at the L2–L3 interspace with persistent right foraminal stenosis. (D) L1 vertebral body. Note more normal appearance of canal.

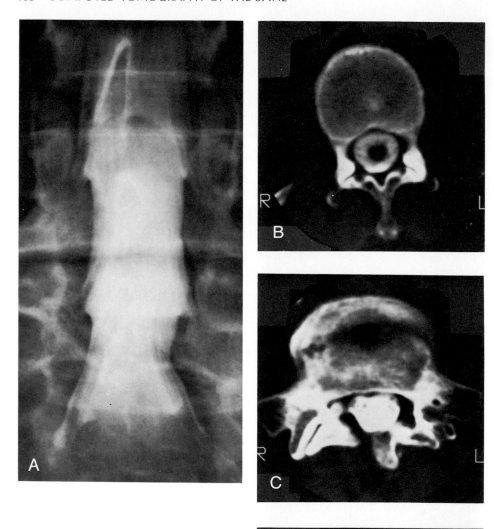

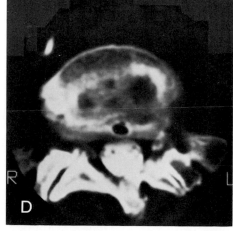

FIG. 8.14 CT in a patient with sciatica and mild lumbar pain and Grade 1 spondylolisthesis L5–S1. (A) Metrizamide myelogram shows an extradural defect. (B) CT with residual metrizamide image of caudal spinal cord which was not well demonstrated myelographically. (C) Observe severe facet abnormalities with ventromedial osteophytic projection from right joint at L5–S1. (D) Note persistence of ostephyte formation with foraminal encroachment and vacuum disc formation immediately caudal to laminectomy site demonstrated above and resolution of lumbar nerve roots within lumbar theca.

the conus medullaris is poorly visualized with metrizamide myelography. For example, in Figure 8.14, CT scanning with remaining myelographic contrast medium defined the distal cord and demonstrated severe facet changes, including medially oriented osteophyte formation, not clearly demonstrated myelographically. Multiple segmental evaluation of spinal stenosis is probably best satisfied myelographically. Gas myelography with hypocycloidal polytomography often affords definition of paramedian canal diameters superior to that obtained with conventional metrizamide myelography; however, the addition of appropriate segmental CT scanning prior to clearance of metrizamide from the subarachnoid space may eliminate this limitation of the positive contrast study.

The relative contribution of previous surgery to degenerative changes of the facet is difficult to establish; however, alteration in force distribution may play a role as in Figure 8.15 in which dramatic facet changes at the site of previous laminectomy were associated with severe foraminal encroachment. Similar severe lateral recess stenosis related to facet hypertrophy persisted after laminectomy in another patient (Fig. 8.16); the inadequacy of laminectomy, not carried through the facet, in decompression of the lateral recesses of this canal is clear. The patient achieved dramatic relief of symptoms with lateral extension of the laminectomy, foraminotomies, and anterior interbody fusion. Pseudospondylolisthesis was present at the L4–L5 level; perhaps the most dramatic lateral and midline stenotic syndromes are seen in association with spondylolisthesis[18] as further evidenced in case Figure 8.17; the contri-

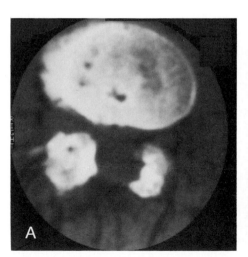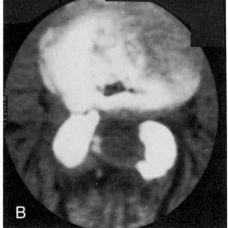

FIG. 8.15   CT in severe lumbar and radiucular pain several years after laminectomy. Note obliteration of extradural fat and marked facet degenerative changes at L3–L4 interspace with marked right foraminal stenosis compounded by vertebral body osteophytic formation. Anteroposterior routine films demonstrated collapse of right interspace with lateral angulation.

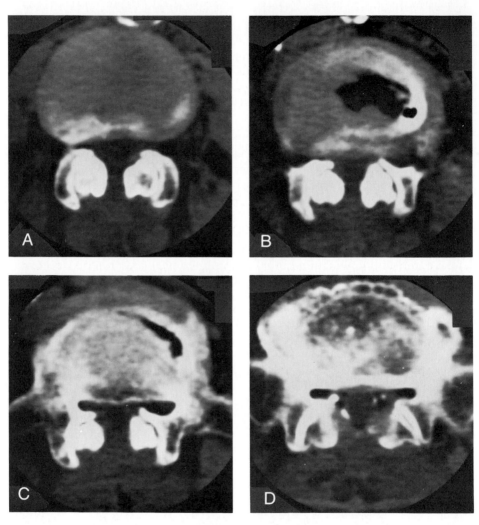

FIG. 8.16 CT of a patient with pseudospondylolisthesis and persistent stenosis after laminectomy for neurogenic claudication. (A) Caudal L3–L4 interspace. Observe narrow laminectomy with persistent foraminal encroachment more marked on the right related to facet hypertrophy. (B) L4–L5 interspace at site of pseudospondylolisthesis. Observe vacuum disc formation and persistent foraminal narrowing despite midline laminar resection. (C,D) L5–S1 interspace. Note severe lateral recess stenosis and radicular displacement related to facet hypertrophy persistent after narrow laminectomy. Relief followed lateral extension of laminectomy and foraminotomies.

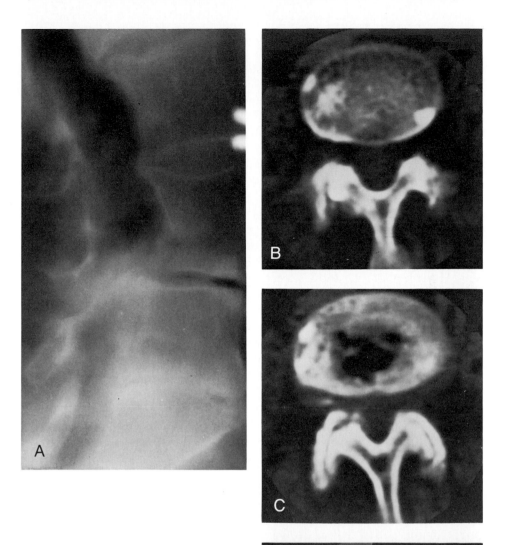

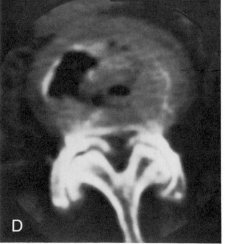

FIG. 8.17 Spondylolisthesis at L4–5 with progressive neurogenic claudication with paraparesis. (A) Polytomographic section of air myelogram. Note spondylolisthesis and virtual absence of gas at L4–L5 level. (B) CT section through caudal L4 vertebral body. Note facet abnormalities. (C) L4–L5 disc. Note vacuum phenomenon and severity of facet changes with right foraminal encroachment. (D) Upper L5 vertebral body. Observe profound stenosis of canal.

bution of soft-tissue elements to stenosis is evident as compressive vectors were difficult to ascertain myelographically. In cases such as these, foraminal exploration may be necessary if adequate surgical decompression is to be accomplished.

CT derived information supplemented myelographic studies and modified clinical management in a case (Fig. 8.18) with traumatic cervical myelopathy. Myelography with both metrizamide and air, coupled with polytomography, demonstrated an increase in the anteroposterior cord diameter with obliteration of anterior and posterior subarachnoid spaces and hence suggested cord edema or hemorrhage or the presence of a laterally situated mass in the spinal canal. CT images supported the latter interpretation and further demonstrated a number of previously unrecognized fractures. Dramatic neurologic improvement was seen after anterior resection of displaced interspace material. Fractures of T12 and L1 led to anterior spinal canal compromise and were associated with marked neurologic deficit in another patient; dorsolateral compression of the canal was most clearly demonstrated by CT scanning (Fig. 8.19). On the basis of this finding, facet resection was carried out in addition to anterior decompression and fusion with excellent myelographic and clinical outcome.

Results of study in patients such as these suggest the possibility of replacement of myelography by CT scanning, however, certain technical limitations must be recalled. Although myelography may effectively evaluate the entire length of the neuraxis, the focus of CT scanning is obligately segmental. Therefore, in cases with epidural metastasis in which multiple deposits may be present and in selected cases of spinal stenosis and degenerative disc disease as noted above, myelographic screening may be necessary. Gantry angle, slice localization, window settings, section thickness, and other technical parameters may assume major importance in demonstration of thin segmental abnormalities (Fig. 8.20). The pyramidial form of thoracic disc prolapse evident in this patient with a Brown–Sequard syndrome dictates the necessity for precise localization and thin sectioning if the apex of the lesion is to be appreciated. Despite the addition of metrizamide to the subarachnoid space, the dimensions of the mass are not readily appreciated with a 5-mm section through the interspace as shown. An exciting field of investigation entails 3-dimensional reconstruction of the spinal canal and may be effective in reduction of such "partial volume" information loss.[12] Artifact related to retained pantopaque or postoperative scarring commonly reduces the utility of CT evaluation in disc disease, as may be seen in Fig. 8.21; with improved resolution and limited use of nonresorbable contrast agents, difficulties of this type may be alleviated.

CT scanning has assumed a legitimate place in the diagnostic armamentarium of craniospinal disorders and may be of value in surgical planning especially in syndromes of lateral canal stenosis related to disc or facet disease processes.[3, 4] Spinal CT scanning may be seen to complement rather than replace myelography and plain films in view of current longitudinal imaging capacities; however, in the patient with single segmental disease, the hazards of myelography may be avoided.

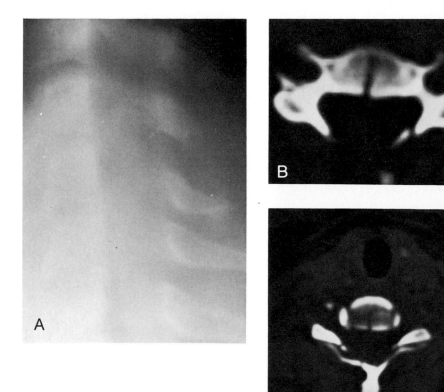

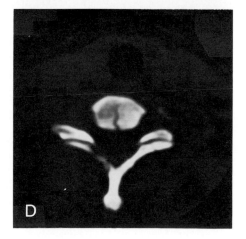

FIG. 8.18 Post-traumatic cervical myelopathy. (A) Polytomographic section of
cervical gas myelography. Note obliteration of anterior and posterior subarachnoid spaces C5 through C7. (B) Anteroposterior vertebral body fracture C5 with
laminar fractures nondisplaced. (C) C6
superior endplate fracture with probable
right herniated nucleus pulposis and laminar fractures. (D) Anteroposterior vertebral body and laminar fractures, C7 vertebral body.

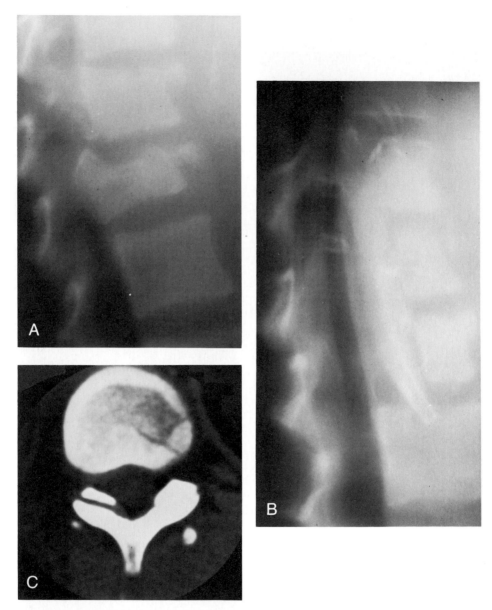

FIG. 8.19 Paraparesis and loss of sphincteric control secondary to T12,L1 fractures. (A) Polytomographic image of air myelogram demonstrates retrodisplacement of fractured L1 vertebral body with canal angulation and stenosis in addition to fracture of the vertebral body of T12. (B) Postoperative study demonstrates adequate decompression. (C–G) CT study in same patient. (C) Note lateral fracture of T11 vertebral body.

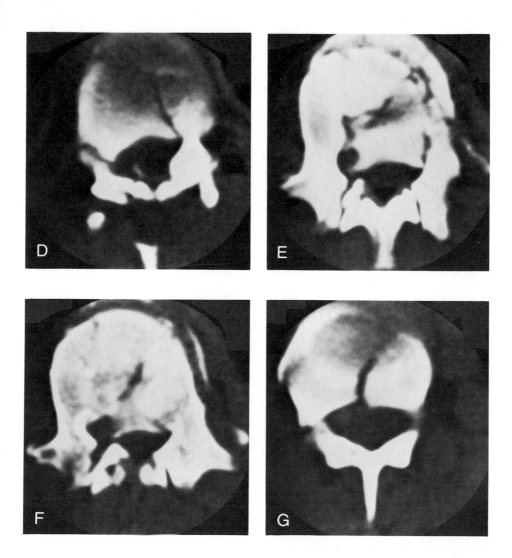

FIG. 8.19 (cont.)   (D) T12 vertebral body fracture involves right pedicle and includes laminar disruption. (E) Extensive disruption of endplate at caudal margin of T12–L1 interspace. (F) At slightly lower levels stenosis of canal is related to retrodisplacement of vertebral body elements and ventromedial facet displacement. (G) Anteroposterior fracture of caudal L1 without distortion of canal.

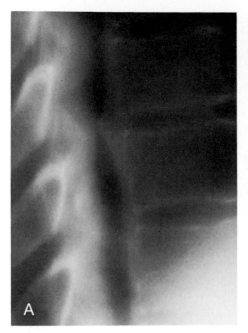

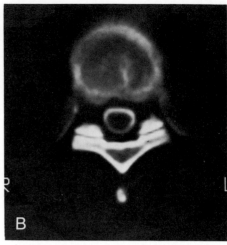

FIG. 8.20 CT and myelography in a thoracic Brown–Sequard Syndrome. (A) Poly-tomographic image obtained at air myelography demonstrates T8–9 disc prolapse with obliteration of anterior subarachnoid space not clearly demonstrated in a 5-mm thick metrizamide enhanced CT section (B).

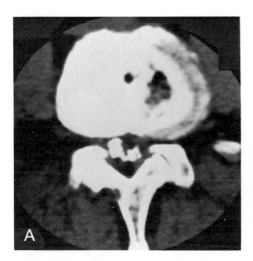

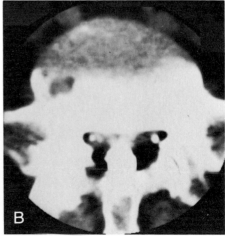

FIG. 8.21 CT artifacts related to laminectomy and retained pantopaque. (A) L4–L5 interspace. Note retained pantopaque and foraminal narrowing related to osteophyte and possible soft-tissue changes. The posterior disc margin is difficult to ascertain with certainty. (B) Retained pantopaque obscures definition of disc boundary at L5–S1.

References

1. Benjamin V, Mangiardi JR, Lin J, Braun I: The value of CT versus conventional myelography in the diagnosis and surgical treatment of lumbar disc disease, American Association of Neurological Surgeons Ann Mtg, Honolulu, Hawaii, April 25–29, 1982, pp. 47–48.

2. Breig A: Biomechanics of the Central Nervous System, Some Basic Normal and Pathologic Phenomena, The Year Book Publishers, Inc., Chicago, 1960.

3. Carrera GF, Haughton VM, Syvertsen A, Williams AL: Computed tomography of the lumbar facet joints. Radiology 134:145–148, 1980.

4. Carrera GF, Williams AL, Haughton VM: Computed tomography in sciatica, Radiology 137:433–437, 1980.

5. de Chiro G, Schellinger D: Computed tomography of spinal cord after lumbar intrathecal introduction of metrizamide (computer-assisted myelography), Radiology 120:101–104, 1976.

6. Durward QJ, Schwiegel JF, Harrison P: Use of the computed tomographic scan in the management of fractures of the thoracic and lumbar spine, Neurosurgery 7(3):289, 1980.

7. Epstein BS, Epstein JA, Jones MC: Lumbar spinal stenosis, pp. 227–239. In Sandrock AR, Ed., The Radiologic Clinics of North America: Symposium on the Spine. WB Saunders Co., Philadelphia, 1977.

8. Hakelius A, Hindmarsh J: The comparative reliability of preoperative diagnostic methods in lumbar disc surgery, Acta Orthop Scand 43:234–238, 1972.

9. Hakelius A, Hindmarsh J: The significance of neurological signs and myelographic findings in the diagnosis of lumbar root compression, Acta Orthop Scand 43:239–246, 1972.

10. Haughton VM, Eldevik OP: Complications from aqueous myelographic media: experimental studies, pp. 183–194. In Sackett JF, Strother CM, Eds., New Techniques in Myelography, Harper & Row, Hagerstown, Maryland, 1979.

11. Haughton VM, Syvertsen A, Williams AL: Soft-tissue anatomy within the spinal canal as seen on computed tomography, Radiology 134:649–655, 1980.

12. Hemmy DC, Herman GT, David DJ: Three-dimensional reconstruction of the spine and skull utilizing computed tomography. American Association of Neurological Surgeons Ann Mtg, Honolulu, Hawaii, April 25–29, 1982, pp. 59–60.

13. Hudgins WR: The predictive value of myelography in the diagnosis of ruptured lumbar discs, J Neurosurg 32:152–162, 1970.

14. Kirkaldy-Willis WH, Heithoff K, Bowen CVA, Shannon R: Pathological anatomy of lumbar spondylosis and stenosis, correlated with the CT scan. pp. 34–55. In Post MJ Donovan, Ed. Radiographic Evaluation of the Spine: Current Advances with Emphasis on Computed Tomography, Masson, New York, 1980.

15. Larson SJ, Sances A, Jr., Walsh PR, Bressler, BC, Hemmy DC: Evoked potentials in neurogenic claudication. 47th Annual Meeting of the American Association of Neurological Surgeons, April 1979, Los Angeles, CA.

16. Mikhael MA, Ciric I, Tarkington JA, Vick NA: Neuroradiological evaluation of lateral recess syndrome, Radiology 140:97–107, 1981.

17. Murphey F: Experience with lumbar disc surgery, Clin Neurosurg 20:1–8, 1973.

18. Newman PH: Stenosis of the lumbar spine in spondylolisthesis, Clin Orthop 115:116–121, 1976.

19. Panjabi MM, White AA: Basic biomechanics of the spine, Neurosurgery 7(1):76–93, 1980.

20. Pennal GF, Schatzker J: Stenosis of the lumbar spinal canal, Clin Neurosurg 18:86–105, 1971.

21. Peterson HO: The hazards of myelography, Radiology 115:237–239, 1975.

22. Ray CD: New techniques for decompression of lumbar spinal stenosis, Neurosurgery 10(5):587–592, 1982.

23. Roaf R: Spinal Deformities. Second Edition. The Pitman Press, Great Britain, 1980.

24. Rothman RH, Campbell RE, Menkowitz E: Myelographic patterns in lumbar disk degeneration, Clin Orthop 99:18–29, 1974.

25. Schmidek HH, Gomes FB, Seligson D, McSherry JW: Management of acute unstable thoracolumbar (T-11-L-1) fractures with and without neurological deficit Neurosurgery 7(1):30–35, 1980.

26. Schneider RC, Crosby EC, Russo RH, Gosch HH: Traumatic spinal cord syndromes and their management, Clin Neurosurg 20:424–492, 1973.

27. Semmes RE: Ruptures of the Lumbar Intervertebral Disc: Their Mechanism, Diagnosis and Treatment, Charles C Thomas, Springfield, IL, 1964.

28. Strother CM: Adverse reactions. pp. 195–202. In JF Sackett and CM Strother, Eds. New Techniques in Myelography. Harper & Row, Hagerstown, Maryland, 1979.

29. Verbiest H: A radicular syndrome from developmental narrowing of the lumbar vertebral canal, J Bone Joint Surg 36B(2):230–237, 1954.

30. Verbiest H: Impending lumbar spondyloptosis. Problems with posterior decompression and foraminotomy: treatment by anterior lumbosacral console fusion, Clin Neurosurg 20:197–203, 1973.

31. Verbiest H: Neurogenic intermittent claudication in cases with absolute and relative stenosis of the lumbar vertebral canal (ASLC and RSLC), in cases with narrow lumbar intervertebral foramina, and in cases with both entities, Clin Neurosurg 20:204–214, 1973.

32. Verbiest H: Pathomorphologic aspects of developmental lumbar stenosis, Orthop Clin No Am 6(1):177–196, 1975.

33. Weinstein PR, Ehni G, Wilson CB: Lumbar spondylosis: diagnosis, management and surgical treatment, Year Book Medical Publishers, Inc., Chicago, 1977.

34. White JC: Results in surgical treatment of herniated lumbar intervertebral discs: investigation of the late results in subjects with and without supplementary spinal fusion—A preliminary report, Clin Neurosurg 13:42–54, 1965.

35. Williams AL, Haughton VM, Syvertsen A: Computed tomography in the diagnosis of herniated nucleus pulposus, Radiology 135:95–99, 1980.

36. Wilson CB, Ehni G, Grollmus J: Neurogenic intermittent claudication, Clin Neurosurg 18:62–85, 1971.

37. Wiltse LL, Kirkaldy-Willis WH, McIvor GWD: The treatment of spinal stenosis, Clin Orthop 115:83–91, 1976.

CASE NO. 1   Johan Johansen

Lumbar Pain

A 31-year-old man with pain in the lower back. The CT scan is at the L5 level, and a window-level for bone is chosen.

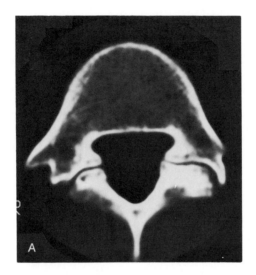

FIGURE 1A

DISCUSSION

There are bilateral clefts in the pars interarticularis indicating spondylolysis. These defects do not represent the facet joints because the slice is not at a disc level. They do not resemble acute fractures because the adjacent bone is sclerotic. The sagittal diameter of the spinal canal is somewhat increased due to a grade 1 spondylolisthesis. CT is very suitable for diagnosing spondylolysis and for showing secondary degenerative changes and bony build-up at the clefts. Although the clinical significance of spondylolysis is not always apparent, CT excludes disc disease as the cause of symptoms.

Final Diagnosis: Spondylolysis with grade 1 spondylolisthesis

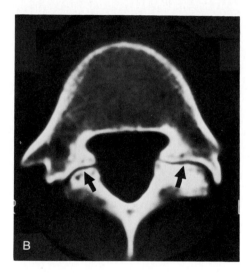

FIGURE 1B   Defects (arrows) in the pars interarticularis.

CASE NO. 2 Johan Johansen

Radicular Pain in Lower Extremity

A 52-year-old man had acute onset of pain radiating to the posterior part of his right leg. The CT scan is at the L5–S1 disc level.

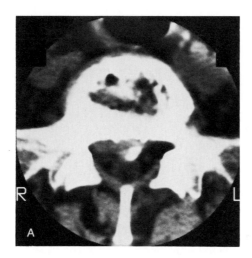

FIGURE 2A

DISCUSSION

The disc is reduced in height resulting in an averaging of disc and end-plate densities, and it contains gas (vacuum phenomenon). There is a posterior localized protrusion of disc substance near the midline on the right side, replacing the normal epidural fat and causing slight posterior displacement of the right S1 root. The CT findings and clinical symptomatology correlate well. Unless compression or displacement of a spinal nerve is demonstrated, a diagnosis of clinically significant disc herniation should not be made in patients with sciatic pain.

Final Diagnosis: Disc degeneration and herniation

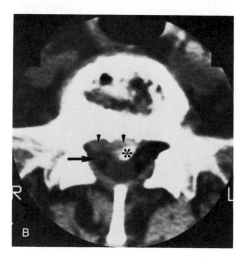

FIGURE 2B Slight posterior displacement of the right S1 root (arrow) due to herniated disc substance (arrowheads). The small area with high density lying medially (asterisk) represents calcification.

CASE NO. 3   Johan Johansen

Radicular Syndrome

A 25-year-old man with right-sided sciatica and hypalgesia suggesting an affection of the L5 nerve root. The CT scan is at the L5–S1 disc level.

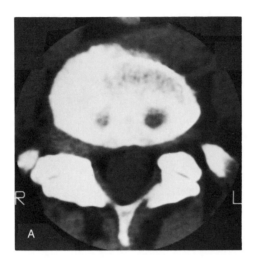

FIGURE 3A

DISCUSSION

On the right side there is a soft-tissue mass behind the disc, filling the intervertebral foramen and completely obscuring the L5 root. These changes are consistent with a lateral disc herniation with compression of the L5 root. A neuroma might be considered in the differential diagnosis. However, there is no enlargement of the intervertebral foramen or any other bony changes.

Final Diagnosis: Lateral disc herniation with compression of nerve root

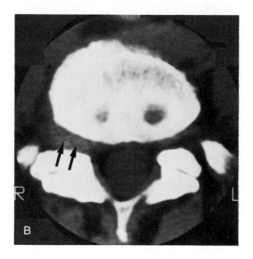

FIGURE 3B Disc material (arrows) filling the right intervertebral foramen and obscuring the nerve root within.

CASE NO. 4   Johan Johansen

Pain in Lower Back and Leg

A 57-year-old man with pain in his lower back and his right leg. The CT scan is at the L4–L5 level.

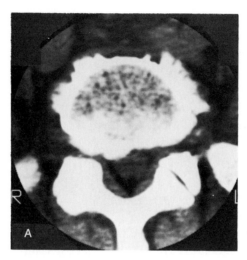

FIGURE 4A

DISCUSSION

There are osteophytes on the lower rim of the L4 vertebral body. A large posterior lateral spur on the right side causes a narrowing of the intervertebral foramen obscuring the fat around the L4 nerve root. This is the probable cause of the patient's symptoms. There are no signs of a disc herniation.

Final Diagnosis: Spondylosis

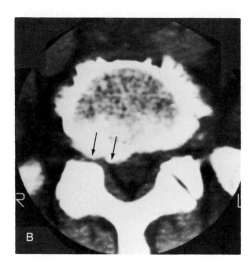

FIGURE 4B   A large osteophyte (arrows) narrows the right intervertebral foramen and causes a slight impression on the dural sac.

CASE NO. 5   Johan Johansen

Lumbar Pain and Radiculopathy

A 72-year-old man with chronic pain in his lower back and both legs, and signs of diffuse bilateral radiculopathy. The CT scan is at the L3–L4 disc level.

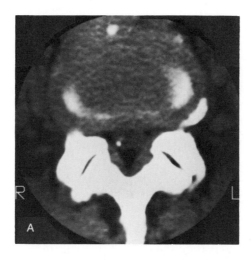

FIGURE 5A

DISCUSSION

There is a generalized protrusion of the disc beyond the margins of the vertebral end-plate, and an osteophytic spur is seen on the left side. The articular processes are hypertrophied, and there is gas in the facet joints (vacuum phenomenon). All these changes contribute to causing a lateral spinal stenosis. The somewhat narrowed and irregular dural sac contains residual droplets of the oily Pantopaque on the right side.

Final Diagnosis: Disc bulging and degenerative facet joints

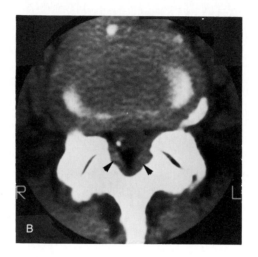

FIGURE 5B   A generalized bulging of the disc and enlargement of the articular processes. The ligamentum flavum is slightly thickened (arrowheads).

CASE NO. 6 Johan Johansen

Radicular Pain in Upper Extremity

A 50-year-old woman with dull ache in her left shoulder and arm, radiating to the first and second digits in her hand. The CT scans at the C5–C6 level were performed following myelography.

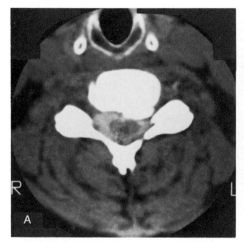
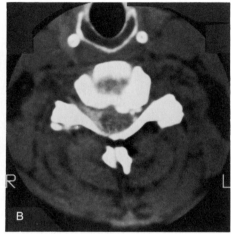

FIGURE 6A   FIGURE 6B

DISCUSSION

There is a large osteophyte at the left posterior lateral margin of C5 causing a narrowing of the C5–C6 intervertebral foramen. There is no contrast filling of the left C6 root sleeve, whereas the right root sleeve is well filled. The osteophyte causes also some impingement on the normal-sized spinal cord, which is well delineated by the intrathecal contrast. The CT changes are consistent with the findings on the myelogram (Fig. 6D), showing a contrast defect in the subarachnoid space corresponding to the area of the left C6 nerve root. In addition, CT excludes a disc herniation.

Final Diagnosis: Nerve root impingement by a large uncinate process osteophyte

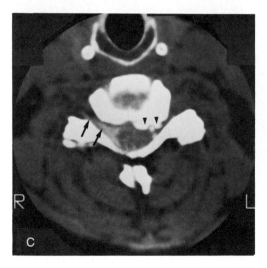

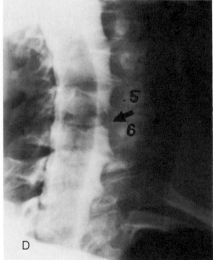

FIGURE 6C   Large uncinate osteophyte (arrowheads) on the left side. Normal contrast-filled root sheath on the right side (arrows).

FIGURE 6D Oblique film from a myelogram of the same patient showing amputation of the left C6 nerve root sheath (arrow).

CASE NO. 7   Johan Johansen

Spinal Trauma

A 41-year-old man sustained a spinal injury from jumping off a bridge. The examination was performed after intrathecal contrast injection.

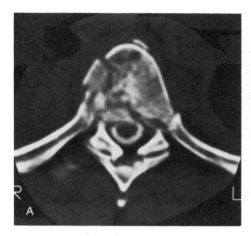

FIGURE 7A   CT scan of T6.

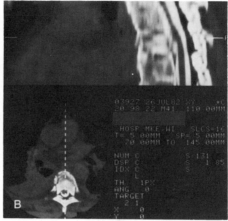

FIGURE 7B   Sagittal reformatting of the spine.

DISCUSSION

There is comminuted compression fracture of T6. A bony fragment is displaced posteriorly on the right side and contacts the spinal cord and partly obliterates the anterior part of the contrast-filled subarachnoid space. The reformatted image reveals that there is in addition a slight posterior displacement of the cord at the fracture level.

Final Diagnosis: Comminuted vertebral fracture

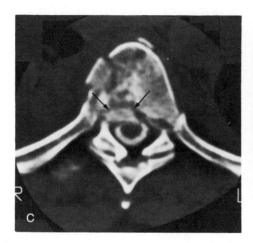 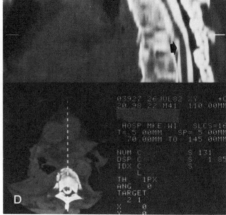

FIGURE 7C A displaced fragment (arrows) compresses the anterior subarachnoid space and contacts the cord.

FIGURE 7D Posterior displacement of the spinal cord (arrow) at the fracture site.

CASE NO. 8 Johan Johansen

Backache and Stiffness

A 52-year-old man with chronic back ache and increasing stiffness. The CT scans are of the L4 lumbar vertebra.

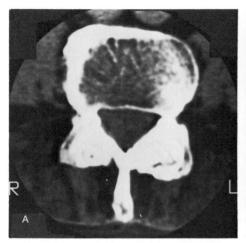

FIGURE 8A

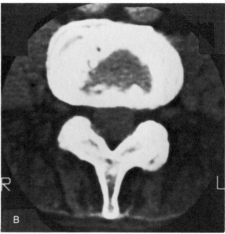

FIGURE 8B

DISCUSSION

The facet joints are completely obliterated, and the articular processes are sclerotic (Fig. 8C). There is calcification in the peripheral rim of the annulus fibrosus and of the anterior longitudinal ligament. These changes are characteristic of ankylosing spondylitis, and the diagnosis is further confirmed by the bony ankylosis found in the sacro-iliac joints (Fig. 8D). Note the atrophic paraspinal muscles. Although the pathologic changes can also be shown on the plain film, CT is very suitable for studying the sacro-iliac and facet joints. *Final Diagnosis:* Ankylosing spondylitis

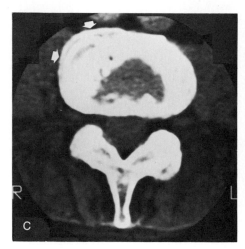 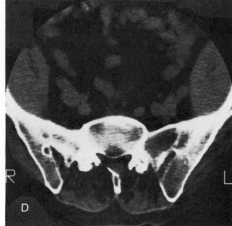

FIGURE 8C Ankylotic facet joints and calcification in the anterior longitudinal ligament (arrows).

FIGURE 8D Ankylosis of the sacro-iliac joints. The changes are most marked on the right side, where there is sclerosis and a posterior erosion.

CASE NO. 9   Johan Johansen

Backache

A 41-year-old man with recurrent ache in his lumbar region. The CT scan is of the L3 vertebra.

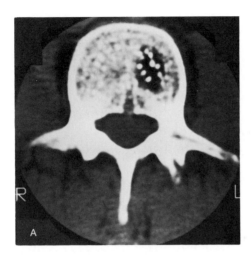

FIGURE 9A

DISCUSSION

On the left side in the vertebral body there is a fairly well demarcated low-density process dotted with small high-density structures that represent sclerotic longitudinal trabeculae. This appearance is characteristic of a hemangioma. The clinical significance of this benign pathologic process is equivocal.

Final Diagnosis: Vertebral hemangioma

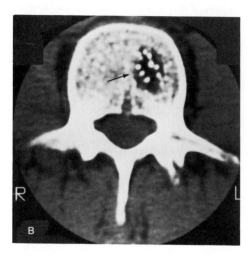

FIGURE 9B Hemangioma in L3 vertebral body (arrow).

CASE NO. 10 Johan Johansen

Buttock Mass and Difficulty in Walking

This 18-month-old girl has a soft indolent mass in the upper medial region of her left buttock. Difficulty in ambulating has been noted. The CT examination was performed after myelography.

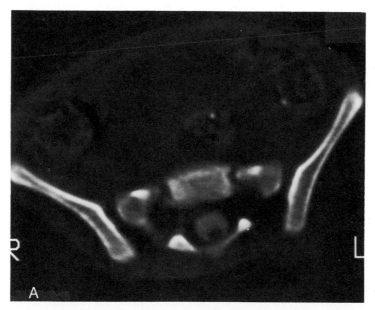

FIGURE 10A   CT scan of the upper sacral region

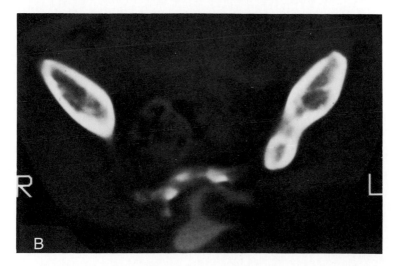

FIGURE 10B   CT scan of the mass in the lower sacral region.

DISCUSSION

Figure 10C shows the spinal cord extending down into the sacral canal. In Figure 10D there is an outpouching of the contrast-filled dural sac through a huge posterior defect in the lower sacrum and in the gluteal muscles. The well-circumscribed and lobulated contrast defect within the expanded dural sac has a very low density of approximately -100 HU consistent with a lipoma. The patient's mass consists of this meningocele and the intradural lipoma. The elongation of the spinal cord and the meningocele are also seen on the myelogram (Fig. 10E), but only CT reveals in addition the true nature and size of the lipoma at the termination of the cord.

Final Diagnosis: Tethered cord and lipomeningocele

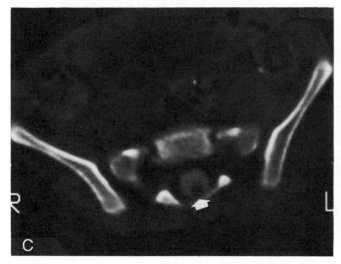

FIGURE 10C   The spinal cord (arrow) extends down to the sacrum.

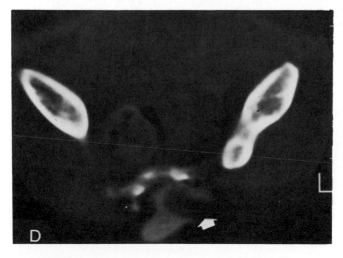

FIGURE 10D   Lipoma within a meningocele.

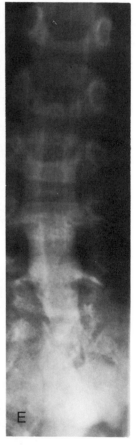

FIGURE 10E   Myelogram showing spinal cord elongation and sacral meningocele.

Index

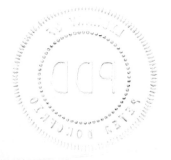

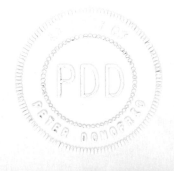